AF229497

Drug-Free Crohn's

DRUG-FREE CROHN'S

Overcoming
Big Doctors, Big Hospitals,
and Big Pharma

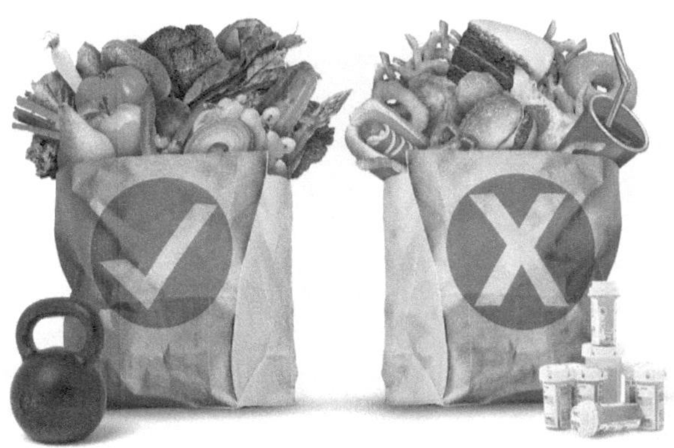

HADLEY OTT

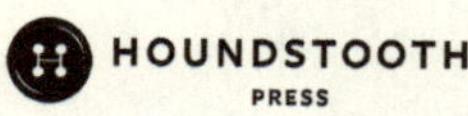

COPYRIGHT © 2026 HADLEY OTT
All rights reserved.

DRUG-FREE CROHN'S
Overcoming Big Doctors, Big Hospitals, and Big Pharma

FIRST EDITION

ISBN   978-1-5445-5053-4 *Hardcover*
        978-1-5445-5052-7 *Paperback*
        978-1-5445-5054-1 *Ebook*

To anyone battling Crohn's disease, ulcerative colitis, or any of the many autoimmune diseases that they were told were incurable. You, too, can become drug-free.

CONTENTS

AUTHOR'S NOTE

Many words are defined throughout this book. They are terms that we use often, but we rarely consider what they actually mean. By reading and defining medical and health terminology, you gain a greater understanding of the healing process and how the body actually works. Many of these definitions come from the *American Heritage Dictionary* (1991 edition). One common frustration for anyone remotely familiar with the American medical system is how technical jargon can be used to confuse patients. I try to avoid this throughout the book. The exception will be when I discuss certain medications—where names cannot be avoided. I must give the disclaimer that I am a medical novice with no formal medical training. I'm not a doctor and have no medical degree. Even as a novice, I was able to research functional medicine and discover how to take charge of my health. I hope to inspire you to do the same.

Secondly, there are some older quotes included that were originally written in a harder-to-understand English, which included words misspelled by modern standards. For clarity, the misspelled words are corrected to their modern spelling. Any mistakes with these words or others are completely my own.

A few well-known individuals in the functional medicine

and alternative healing world are mentioned in this book. Their names are not altered. However, the names of physicians who I personally dealt with have been changed. If there are real-life physicians who share these made-up names, it is entirely coincidental.

Finally, the Bible verses quoted all come from the New Revised Standard Version (NRSV).

INTRODUCTION

For nearly fifteen years, I struggled with Crohn's disease. After being diagnosed at the age of twelve, I took numerous medications and underwent a number of tests and procedures—all while dealing with the same symptoms. But all that has changed. After running the medical gauntlet, which included dangerous biologic drugs and an irreversible surgery, I finally healed myself naturally. I want anyone with an autoimmune disease, including Crohn's, to experience the liberating feeling that comes with being drug-free.

After going down the rabbit hole of functional medicine in an effort to cure myself, I feel qualified to give you the basics so you can start living well. In addition to my insights and research, a critique of common hospital and doctor practices will be discussed. This brings to mind a crucial point: Most doctors don't have the illness you are experiencing. What better way to learn than from someone who has overcome these challenges themselves?

Being healthy is the natural state. Most humans are not born sick and are not intended to live a life structured with medical appointments, or to be tethered to the pharmacy and their prescriptions. Man is meant to live life to the fullest. He is to be fit, active, creative, and robust. Theodore Roosevelt's call to live the strenuous life was nothing more than an order to be true to the instinctive human condition—a call for men to exhaust the energy within themselves, becoming unshakeable physical specimens in the process.

Throughout history, living a healthy lifestyle and eating a proper diet came naturally. There was no other option but organic food. Only whole fruits and vegetables and wild game could be consumed in the absence of processing and modern preserving methods. With no fast-food restaurants, a man had to kill a deer, pick berries, or catch a fish if he wanted supper. Man's work—as a farmer, carpenter, stone mason, or tanner—ensured his body would receive exercise and his muscles would show definition. Hence, there weren't many fat pioneers or pilgrims.

This is not to paint an ideal picture of human existence before the modern era. Hardly. There were epidemics, wars, barbaric medical treatments, and an ignorance of germs that accounted for many premature deaths. Around the year 1500 AD, approximately one in three people died before turning five.[1] Life was hard, no doubt, but many of the chemicals, toxins, and preservatives that plague Americans' diets today were lacking in earlier times.

The Industrial Revolution changed civilization forever. Life expectancy tripled within two centuries of America's founding,[2] and we now enjoy a host of luxury goods. But these advancements have come at a cost, as our food and lifestyle have deteriorated in the process. In earlier times, the diet may have been ideal to reach old age, but a simple infection or a battle wound received in younger years, combined with ignorance in treating the ailment, ended life prematurely. In the old days, people had the proper diet, but not the medicine. Today we have the medicine to enable old age, but not the diet to do it naturally.

America now has the medical knowledge and technology to ensure more people live longer, but these are often just corrections of previous errors that enable longevity. Doctors now wash their hands before delivering a baby, and serious bodily injuries now stand a greater chance than ever before of being successfully treated. Lifesaving surgeries are now available for those in horrific accidents. Still, Americans are increasingly sick and often chronically ill. It begs the question of how we got here and whether previous generations were aware of their physical well-being.

Those in Colonial America were noticeably healthier than their cousins in Europe.[3] The fresh atmosphere; hardships on the frontier; the absence of large, dirty cities; and the rugged spirit of liberty and individualism contributed to a population that lived longer and grew taller than those in the Old World.[4] This country's frontier produced a healthy lot of men with the strength and determination to conquer the continent.

By contrast, Americans today are overweight, increasingly sick, less ambitious, and more sedentary than ever before. Why is this happening? In short, the natural state has been corrupted by a host of man-made substances.

Over the last century, and more notably in the last four decades, an increasing amount of chemicals, toxins, and additives have been added to our food supply and environment. Some 194 million Americans now suffer from at least one chronic health condition.[5] RFK Jr.'s presidential run in 2024 brought this issue to the forefront. People began checking labels, exploring regenerative agriculture, and questioning whether they should be taking their medications or receiving an upcoming vaccine.

This book, however, is not about the food industry, per se, or the harmful substances that have been added to our diet and environment. It is, rather, a story of the effects, notably the autoimmune diseases exacerbated by these and other factors. Crohn's disease is one of more than one hundred known auto-immune diseases, and more than two million Americans have some form of IBD, including Crohn's.[6] Some thirty thousand people are diagnosed every year with Crohn's.[7] Conventional medicine has failed to treat autoimmune diseases, including Crohn's. The medical establishment and pharmaceutical indus-try would have you believe that prescription drugs, doctor's appointments, and routine tests are needed to manage these conditions, but they can never be cured. As a result, patients are inundated with the dreadful notion that they are sick for life.

I contend that not only is Crohn's disease treatable, but it is also curable and preventable in many cases—but not with conventional doctors, hospitals, and medicines. You can over-come Crohn's or any autoimmune disease you are struggling with, but it will require a different approach. This book serves as a testament that it can be done.

I have gone through the wringer of conventional doctors, hospitals, and Big Pharma. Having experienced it all—from biologic drugs to surgery—and still finding no relief, I decided to trust my gut and take a leap of faith. I quit my doctors and medicine and healed myself naturally using guidance from functional medicine providers and tailored supplements, along with fitness and nutrition. Above all, I strongly contend that there is a spiritual component to healing. Indeed, an entire chapter is devoted to the power of prayer and the guidance God gives us in the Bible to become the healthiest versions of our-selves. My Christian faith was paramount in finally overcoming this "incurable" disease and becoming drug-free. Whether your faith in Jesus is strengthened by your health challenges, or you find Christianity in the depths of your physical suffering, you cannot ignore the incredible power that comes from asking God to heal you.

Nutrition, fitness, and faith can heal you. It requires more effort, more focus, and more discipline than the convenience of taking medications. But the results are worth it. Besides, the secular modern approach has proven to be financially wasteful and ineffective.

Trillions of government dollars have been spent on health care in the US in recent decades, with a portion of that money going toward researching cures for chronic diseases such as Crohn's, diabetes, and more profound illnesses such as cancer. In 2023, the United States collectively spent $4.9 trillion on health care, or $14,570 per person.[8] Health care spending in 2023 accounted for more than 17 percent of the GDP,[9] representing a significant share of the American economy. Despite the massive influx of cash and resources thrown at health problems, our outcomes have been getting worse. Some six in ten American adults suffer from at least one chronic health problem, while over 40 percent of people have at least two.[10] Americans are taking an increasing amount of prescription drugs. In early 2025, 68 percent of Americans were on at least one prescription medication. A quarter of the population was on four or more prescriptions.[11] This is not normal, and it's not working.

When it comes to autoimmune diseases, including Crohn's and colitis, researchers are looking for Camelot in their quest to find a cure. While one may exist, a far greater hope lies in noninvasive functional medicine. That is, addressing the root causes of your illness and preventing future episodes altogether—discovering *why* you are sick and then customizing a plan to treat yourself and achieve lasting health.

That is what this book is about: having the confidence to take charge of your own body and heal yourself naturally.

This book is not a medical textbook. It's not even a self-help book—which can carry the connotation of some irredeemable flaw you have as a person. Not at all! Your health challenges don't make you any less of a person, but they can serve as a rite of passage to a better and healthier version of yourself. This book is the starting point and a call to reject the conventional medical advice you've received. Imagine Crohn's or other health problems you face to be a wall in the house of your life that needs to come down. The decision has been made: It's time for a remodel. This book is the hammer, and its pages are the first swing. We'll make a dent, and the wall will know it's coming down. Depending on the severity of your autoimmune disease, this book alone may be sufficient to get you well—or you may require further work to finally get there. I pray the success of this first book will offer me the opportunity to write a second one—a more in-depth volume on how to, step by step, treat every symptom you are suffering from. Right now, the most important thing for you to understand is this: It is possible to heal yourself naturally *and* thrive. Whether you have Crohn's, ulcerative colitis, or other chronic and autoimmune diseases, I hope you will be inspired to take agency over your own body and health.

This book has been written for anyone suffering from an autoimmune disease or chronic medical condition that they were told was incurable, particularly men. Crohn's causes embarrassing symptoms, creates immense insecurity, and can prevent men from living their most productive lives. Men are supposed to be doers and risk-takers. But these health challenges can hold us back. It is especially important that young men with autoimmune disease adhere to these insights. I don't want you to hold yourself back as I did during my crucial formative years. If you are diagnosed with Crohn's or colitis at a young age, I want you to heal yourself naturally and reject the precept of being sick for life.

It is my great hope and prayer to provide you with the encouragement and inspiration to realize that you have agency over your own body, that you can become the healthiest, most active version of yourself. You, too, can live your life without any constraints imposed by physicians or hospital mandates. You, too, can become drug-free.

PART ONE

FLAWS IN THE SYSTEM

Chapter One

IS THIS FOR LIFE?

"Every problem has in it the seeds of its own solution."
—NORMAN VINCENT PEALE

One rule I believe men should live by is this: Don't be a self-revealer. Unfortunately, this maxim of mine will be heavily violated in the following chapter. However, it is necessary that you understand my own journey in order for me to help you with yours.

Stomach issues seemed to always plague me during my childhood, which resulted in many trips to the doctor and the school nurse. As a second grader in 2005, I had severe diarrhea and incontinence issues, a painful anal fistula, and my body was skeletally skinny. My bones showed through my skin, and I was likened to an Ethiopian. I saw my first gastroenterologist, or GI doctor, and through the course of a year, enough blood was drawn to fill a milk jug.

The same year, my father was deployed to Iraq, and worrying became routine. My mother and grandmother speculated that there could be a connection between my worrying as a seven-year-old and the dreadful symptoms I was experiencing. During July of that year, I had my first colonoscopy and endoscopy: A small camera attached to a pencil-thin rod was inserted into my backside, while another tube was stuck down my throat. I didn't know what the doctors were looking for, or what it would mean if they found it. Thankfully, nothing was found, and I eventually returned to a "normal" condition. Whether it was my father coming home, or the symptoms just disappearing on their own, it remains a mystery how I ever overcame this awful season.

Despite the pain and discomfort, this episode did little to curtail my diet, and I quickly resumed my old eating habits.

I grew up eating the Standard American Diet (SAD). Many of you are likely familiar and probably grew up consuming the majority of your calories from these foods as well. I was an enthusiast for ultra-processed junk food: chips, pretzels, candy, eater-snacks—you name it. Fast food, chicken tenders, ice cream, desserts of any kind, cereals, Cokes—I could devour them all. To be sure, we ate fruit and vegetables. Generally, vegetables meant a salad with bacon bits and Thousand Island dressing. Eating fruit meant canned peaches or fresh watermelon in the summer. A healthy school lunch was deli turkey on white bread, chips, cookies, and applesauce.

I was somewhat active, but I did not move nearly as much as young boys are supposed to. With my gluttonous appetite and lack of exercise, I became rather portly compared to the skin-and-bones version of myself that existed just a few years earlier. Not only was I portly, but there also wasn't a trace of muscle on me. I could barely do push-ups or other simple body-weight exercises.

As my elementary school days progressed, I changed schools for the fourth and fifth grades, which was customary in my district. However, as I prepared for the fifth grade, a depressed state overtook me. In August 2008, I had the desire to end my life and planned on avoiding water until I dropped dead of thirst. I was miserable in public school and completely out of place with my contemporaries. That year was not easy, but I made it through. It's no coincidence that exactly one year later, I once again began getting sick—very sick. It was a vile spell that nearly killed me, even if I had somewhat overcome those hellish thoughts of expiring myself. Those thoughts lingered, but there were no active attempts for the next few years.

These three factors that culminated at this time—poor diet, poor mood, and no exercise—contributed, I'm certain, to the near-fatal bout with Crohn's disease just a year later. A combination of a poor diet and a poor mindset made me sick, which is why the two must be addressed. It's not enough to have a clear mind and healthy thoughts if your diet is a mess, and vice versa. Nor can you neglect exercise even when your diet is great. In the course of your own healing, keep these points in mind. Now, here's how I got Crohn's.

During the summer of 2009, I began to experience more symptoms of bowel discomfort, stomach pain, and frequent bathroom trips. As the dog days of summer waned, my body began to shrivel. It was not the heat and sweat or vigorous exercise responsible for the weight loss—I hardly had the energy for that. By the start of school in August, it became a common occurrence for me to throw up after eating. I could hardly keep food down, and my stomach was hurting.

My grandfather turned eighty on August 12, 2009, my first day of the sixth grade. The first day of school was always a half-day. My mother picked me up and took us out to eat—a special thing she always did on the first and last days of school. This was an occasion I usually looked forward to, but on this day, I dreaded it. We ate roast beef sandwiches and curly fries at Arby's. I wasn't hungry, but I still couldn't shake my stubborn childhood tendency to never turn down food.

As soon as I made it home, I threw up everything I had eaten and felt terrible. Worse, we hosted a party for my grandfather that evening with family I would normally be glad to see, and with lots of food I would normally love to eat—barbeque, potatoes, chips, cake, ice cream, and more. Of course, I tried eating and felt worse for it. The stomach pain and vomiting persisted, and I gradually lost my appetite in the months that followed. By October and November, eating anything caused such sharp stomach pains that I rejected food altogether.

As a twelve-year-old in November of that year, I was four foot nine and fifty-three pounds. Most girls in my class weighed twice as much as I did.

THE DIAGNOSIS

As I approached gastrointestinal Armageddon, I attended a field trip to the Adventure Science Center in Nashville. This is normally an incredible place to visit and tons of fun when you're young. Among the activities we were allowed to do was a spacewalk simulation, which let us experience the effects of zero gravity. The bad news for me was that you had to weigh at least eighty pounds to participate. I failed to make weight and was only allowed to complete the simulation typically reserved for elementary school-aged kids. I ate a few crackers for lunch, but the sharp stomach pains continued.

This may sound too naive in hindsight, but even though eating was causing stomach pain, vomiting, and severe diarrhea, we knew of nothing else to do. I continued to try different foods and just hoped for a better outcome on my insides.

I have a great family, but they never understood the proper way to eat. They were not foodaholics by any means, but they weren't CrossFit athletes either. We thought our diet was reasonably healthy. Still, if cheese was being served, you were expected to eat it, and they would give you a hard time for your refusal to eat foods that made you feel bad or foods you simply didn't like. At a young age, most of us lack credibility among the grown-ups in our lives, and they don't take us seriously when we say our stomachs hurt.

Stomach aches are often viewed by grown-ups as a cop-out for a young kid. Throwing up was viewed as creating a disgusting mess to clean up (and of course it is). What's often ignored is that these are symptoms of something wrong internally, specifically within the digestive tract. My symptoms got worse and were largely neglected to the point where I was withering away. I was probably a few weeks—if not days—away from dying altogether.

My local doctor in Clarksville was unable to explain what was happening and, out of desperation, I was taken to Vanderbilt Children's Hospital just days before Thanksgiving. I was given an IV and soon had an MRI done. The GI doctor who reviewed the results said it looked like Crohn's disease, but I was to come back in a few days for a colonoscopy to confirm his suspicions. He had a very indifferent personality, but we knew nothing other than trusting the doctor's judgment. Although I could eat very little, he said the food at home was better than at the hospital, so I might as well go back home for the next few days. The irony, of course, was that I couldn't eat that much in the first place, no matter how good my mother's food was.

While there during my first stay, I'll never forget the expression on the face of a doctor when I told her that I had ordered and eaten chicken strips from the hospital's cafeteria. The other doctors had already insisted that food had nothing to do with my condition, and maybe this doctor believed the dogma herself. Yet something on her face gave away an instinctive understanding that food had everything to do with it, whether she was allowed to admit it or not.

We returned days later for a week-long stay. In my absolute frailest state, I underwent a colonoscopy without much incident. But this procedure did confirm the existence of Crohn's disease. I was placed on prednisone (a steroid medication) and a feeding tube, which I continued for about a month. Feeding tubes are used for patients who are either unable to eat, or whose bodies are too weak to handle solid foods. Having the tube inserted was about the worst experience I can remember, but I was too weak to resist. Bedridden, my head was elevated by a couple of nurses. Without warning, a tube was shoved up my nose, and I gagged as the device passed the nasal cavity and entered the back of my throat.

I did not eat the day before or the day of the colonoscopy. Nor did I eat on the days that followed. In all, I went five days without a single bite of food. When I finally broke the extended Crohn's-induced fast, I got to enjoy some Teddy Grahams (another unhealthy option!). I still remember how bad it hurt my teeth to chew after such a long hiatus.

Once my stomach pain was under control, I was discharged from the hospital. The doctors loaded me up on pills, and I took a handful every day for several months thereafter. I couldn't tell you what the purpose of any of those pills was, other than prednisone. I was told to take them, so I did. I always wondered what the plastic cases with seven little doors on my grandparents' bathroom counter were for, and now I knew. They were pill boxes, and I had my own to rival them.

The feeding tube was removed just a few days before Christmas. Although I could eat while using the device, it tugged at my throat each time I swallowed. I was grateful to have it out, but it would soon become part of my daily life again. In addition to the pills and feeding tube, another aspect of my doctor-prescribed routine was a low-residue diet. This entailed avoiding raw fruits and vegetables, nuts, seeds, and other foods high in fiber. It sounded (and still sounds) completely counterproductive. To get healthy, I must avoid healthy foods and instead eat processed grains that I was told were easier for my stomach to handle and digest.

Still, when your body is recovering from a nearly fatal medical emergency, you have to make health compromises and allow your body to heal. It doesn't mean you eat processed food forever—only until your body has recovered. Another way to think about it is to consider that walking is healthy, and sitting is less so. But if your leg is broken, you have to sit until your body has recovered so you can be healthy enough to walk again.

By 2010, I was weaned off prednisone and went on a feeding tube full time. This was a difficult process to learn, but I managed to become pretty good at it; that is, putting the tube down my throat every evening then hooking the other end to a pump that infused four cans of who-knows-what into my stomach. Strangely, this act (and, in my judgment, my remarkable ability to complete it) gave me a tremendous sense of accomplishment. Even better, I was starting to exercise and made it my goal to achieve six-pack abs.

While in the hospital in December 2009, I watched a Navy football game on the TV in my room. I immediately became a fan of the Midshipmen. The old-school triple option offense fascinated me. Ken Niumatalolo became my favorite coach and Kriss Proctor my favorite quarterback. If there was one player I idolized, it was Navy's star fullback Alex Teich. I'll never forget his 2011 touchdown run against Army in which he dove for the end zone. He was big, fast, strong, and athletic. Moreover, his very presence at the Naval Academy immediately conveyed intelligence as well as a great demeanor, strong work ethic, and patriotism. I wanted to be him.

Lying there in a hospital bed in my absolute weakest state, I was determined to somehow get my body in shape. I had no guidance, but basic intuition told me just to get outside and move. I became more physically active than ever before in the months following my release. By late spring 2010, I was walking around my neighborhood and playing basketball in the driveway and football in the yard. With the goal of building core strength and toning my abs, I started using some light weights my mother had. I began doing a host of ab exercises and push-ups. Thousands of crunches and sit-ups were soon performed weekly. At that point, I started to feel good for a change and better about myself. As I progressed in my daily regimen of calisthenics, another football player caught my attention, Herschel Walker. Although Walker's playing days were long over, I was inspired by his childhood story of transforming his body through the same means I was attempting to use.

For the duration of my seventh-grade year, I subsisted largely on a nightly feeding tube diet. Any traditional eating I was doing, as my doctors explained, was only for fun. The cans of awful-smelling yellow stuff dripping into my stomach each night were sufficient for growth, they said. Of course, I still ate some, but my nutritional consciousness had not yet developed. So, when I did eat, it was often still the same junk. Throughout that academic year, I spent most of my lunch breaks in the school library—reading while my classmates dined.

The feeding tube worked well until September 2011, when I was hospitalized again. Following a recent bout of pain and other symptoms, I was driven to Vanderbilt by my father on my birthday. My stomach pain could be severe at times, but it was not excessive. Nevertheless, the doctors determined that the feeding tube no longer worked, and I faced the possibility of resorting to biologics.

The scary-sounding term "biologics" refers to medications and medical treatments that use genetic material of other animals in the production process and in the product itself. Remicade was the drug my doctors were eager to start me on. My parents had wise and well-founded reservations. For one, Remicade increases your risk for cancer. According to my doctor (in 2011), the odds of getting cancer were about two in one thousand. I now know that the actual odds were and are much higher—anecdotally, we all know this to be true. (Most people probably have fewer than one thousand people in their family and social circle, and yet know multiple people who have gotten cancer.) But at the time, the great fear was that Remicade doubled this seemingly small risk to four in one thousand.

ALTERNATIVES

At some point in 2010, prior to my second major hospital stay, I also began seeing a physician of alternative medicine—Dr. Harrow (name changed), a man with crazy hair. His practice was more tailored to patients, as his recommendations were based on blood tests and other metrics. I began taking supplements, including fish oil and an awful-tasting health drink. At the time, I remember it tasting like dirt, but it was probably the healthiest thing for me. Moreover, he provided a list of the only foods that should be eaten. These were foods from the earth—raw, organic, and natural. His list included a host of vegetables, fruits, and grains, some of which I had never heard of, including quinoa. His recommendations also called for weekly acupuncture treatments.

Acupuncture is an ancient Chinese method of using strategic needle pricks for reducing pain and inflammation. Originally, the needles were made of bamboo. As blacksmithing improved, metal needles were eventually employed. My hesitation to get stuck with needles yet again quickly vanished after the first appointment. The needles were as thin as hair, and with a gentle tap, the acupuncturist inserted the needles into the surface of my skin. Needles were tapped on my arms, legs, chest, and stomach. Then his assistant connected a select number of carefully chosen needles to a machine that sent an electric pulse throughout my body. Acupuncture is an unusual and slightly uncomfortable procedure, yet I found it relaxing and soothing.

A cousin whose son experienced stomach problems years earlier had a book called *Patient Heal Thyself* by Dr. Jordan Rubin. This was an especially meaningful book as the author suffered from Crohn's disease as a young college student and relates his experience. Incredibly, despite all of the doctors, treatments, and medicines, nothing worked for the young Rubin. Practically out of desperation, he turned to a man in California who vowed he could be cured with the proper nutrition. Through his book, I was immersed in the role food plays in our health and inspired by Rubin's ability to heal himself. It left an impression that has stuck with me.

I launched a half-hearted effort to implement the teachings of Dr. Harrow and Dr. Rubin. Busy schedules and obligations, to say nothing of the job it takes to find, procure, and prepare these foods, made it very difficult to go all-in. My parents were still curious enough to see what the doctors had to say about *Patient Heal Thyself.* The reaction was telling, and a bit insulting. It was immediately dismissed on the grounds that the impact of nutrition and diet on Crohn's had not been studied. (An obvious follow-up should have been *Why not?!*) I have since learned that medical schools either offer no nutritional classes or offer very few, and they are not required.

Still, it seems I couldn't escape the prospect of getting put on Remicade. I'll never forget the reaction of my female gastroenterologist, Dr. McDowell, as these points were being made. She was a nice enough lady, personally. Nevertheless, she took on the persona of a prison guard leading a condemned man to his execution—without a bit of sympathy for the inmate. Her body language and expression gave it away. *I'm putting you on Remicade. Yes, it doubles your risk of cancer. And there's nothing you can do about it.*

In hindsight, an important lesson was learned that will be fleshed out in other chapters: Trust your intuition. When something doesn't seem right, it probably isn't. When something sounds wrong, it probably is.

My doctor ended the feeding tube treatment, and the decision was made to put me on Remicade. This was a scary drug for my parents and me, but none of us knew what else to do. In what may be considered a remarkable run, I remained on Remicade from the fall of 2011 through the fall of 2018 largely without incident. Although nothing major that would merit a hospital stay occurred, there were always persistent symptoms flirting with me. I never grew quite like my contemporaries, and I lived through the cream of my youth with this dreadful concept in me: *You are sick for life.*

Things would take a turn during the fall of my junior year at UT Martin. Following a very stressful semester of school and work, I went to the emergency room after a Christmas party in December. I had been feeling bad in the weeks leading up to the incident and lost my appetite for food and exercise. There were several moments late in the semester when I had significant stomach pain, and it was especially difficult trying to study and take finals with an upset stomach. Somehow, I managed to pass with all A's. I ate very little at the Christmas party, despite the temptation of the seasonal delicacies. Soon after I got home from the gathering, I was bent over in pain on the floor of my room. Rounds of throwing up followed. *What are you throwing up?!* I thought. *You've hardly eaten anything in days!*

Late at night, my mother drove me—for the umpteenth time—to Vanderbilt Children's Hospital (yes, I was getting too old for this place). In the course of my experience with Crohn's, I developed a pretty high tolerance for pain. But the stomach pain I felt that night—December 22, 2018—was awful, truly the worst of anything I've ever experienced with Crohn's. I was on death's door, it seemed. There were a few young residents who were anxious to operate on me right then, but thankfully, my symptoms were quickly resolved with the use of steroids. At that moment, stopping the pain was my only priority. An MRI revealed I had a stricture, or scarred tissue, on a portion of my intestines. This stricture became tight, preventing food from passing through. My age made my presence more than awkward to the staff, who were all expecting a slow time anyway on account of Christmas.

The nurses wanted to insert a large tube through my nose in order to pump out any remaining food inside me. My experience with the feeding tube years earlier came in handy, and I inserted the tube myself—to the amazement of the nurses present. This was done to relieve the stomach pain but also to prep my colon in the event of emergency surgery. The doctors were still eager to operate, and a surgical team consisting of a short Indian fellow, an annoying female Michigan grad, and a pudgy older male surgeon made multiple trips to my room, hoping I was ready for the scalpel. Thankfully they weren't needed.

Despite a quick recovery, I was again placed on the low-residue diet. This was practically a white flour diet, consisting of no vegetables and virtually no fruit. Again, it is very ironic that this was considered "healthy" for me. While subsisting on the diet recommended by my doctors, I gained weight during the spring semester. In the meantime, the long-awaited transition to the adult hospital was made, and Dr. Morris placed me in the tender care of Dr. Horne.

THE NUCLEAR OPTION

The nuclear option, or surgery, was still on the table, and the doctors were pressing hard in favor of it. In fact, all roads were leading to surgery as long as I stayed with Vanderbilt. I had managed to recover from my December spell okay, but it was heavily contingent on the diet I was on. A couple of appointments were made with a surgeon, and momentum was all on the side of operating. After appointments with my new doctor and the surgeon, the decision was made to remove the stricture in my intestine, despite my heavy reservations and a great deal of naivety about the procedure itself. The primary argument in favor of removing the stricture at that time was that it could be done in a controlled environment, not in a chaotic, emergency fashion with whoever happened to be at the hospital when the surgery suddenly became urgent. It also reduced the risk of my surgeon needing to create a stoma and my having to live with an ileostomy bag. Moreover, my surgeon would perform the operation laparoscopically, which is minimally invasive. Instead of a foot-long vertical scar, I would have a few inch-long scars—a reasonable trade-off, I guess.

Prior to the operation, I consulted an old family friend who had practiced general surgery for more than thirty years. He assured me that the removal of a stricture was "straightforward surgery" and there was really no need to worry. I was grateful for his input.

In July 2019, the "minimally invasive" operation was performed, leaving five scars—one for each incision. I quickly realized that movie characters who are wounded in the gut and keep going are either a heck of a lot tougher than me, or it's just pure Hollywood fiction. I could not have imagined how difficult it would be just to try and sit up, much less walk, following this operation. But the human body is remarkable, and within a few days I was back up and walking quite well. Within two months, the feeling that I had been operated on finally passed. Unless you've experienced it firsthand, you might be unaware of the eerie, weak feeling that lingers post-surgery. I couldn't wait to get over that.

After the surgery, I continued my Remicade infusions. In general, it seems the trend is for doctors to prescribe drugs (drugs that don't actually *cure* you) for as long as they can until they resort to the big money-maker: surgery. Then they resume the drugs and repeat the process for the rest of your lives. I wanted a way out of this rut, but I lacked the confidence to speak up and find my own way.

With the benefit of hindsight and a greater understanding of functional medicine, I would have skipped surgery and opted instead to use the elemental diet, which gives the intestines a rest by replacing solid food with a series of drinks—nutritional powder mixed with water. This diet can be followed for weeks, even months if needed. Such a break from solid food can allow the body to heal itself and avoid the permanent damage done by surgery. Greater detail on the wonders of the elemental diet will come in a later chapter.

Once my bowels reactivated, I began losing a lot of weight and ultimately lost some forty pounds by the end of the summer. (Talk about summer weight loss!) The weight loss had its advantages though. Upon returning to UT Martin for my senior year, I began exercising in the mornings and performing various calisthenics when the gym opened at 6:00 a.m. If the surgery had any benefit, it allowed me to achieve physical feats that always eluded me. For the first time in my life, despite years of training, I was able to complete pull-ups regularly. In August, I began doing pull-ups in the morning, three at a time, three times a week. In late November, I completed a workout in which I performed 550 pull-ups in about two hours. The final five reps were done with a forty-five-pound weight attached to my waist. I weighed around 155 pounds and finally achieved the washboard abs I spent a decade pursuing. My health had never been better, it seemed. My confidence improved too. In July, I was too weak to even raise my head. Four months later, I was doing the hardest upper-body exercise at an elite level.

Heading into the spring semester, my fitness and health were in check, and I was feeling good about myself. Then COVID-19 hit.

LOCKDOWN

I have wondered if most people experienced what I did during the lockdowns. When schools were closed in March 2020, I instantly lost most of my friends in addition to my favorite outlet, the gym. With the gym closed, and grocery stores facing constant shortages, my fitness level dropped significantly. Once your body has grown acclimated to lifting weights, it becomes difficult to maintain your progress and strength on bodyweight exercises alone.

Moreover, summer was rapidly approaching. I was about to graduate college with a 3.95 GPA, *summa cum laude*, and yet I had zero job prospects. Despite the health challenges I faced, I hold myself fully accountable for failing to be more proactive in this regard. It was my very naive assumption that I could easily parlay decent grades into a job whenever I wanted. Many who graduated with inferior grades were quickly employed in professional positions, while I took an entry-level job at Walmart just to stay busy in the weeks after school ended.

An important lesson was learned: A good job—or anything worth having in life—is not going to fall into your lap. You must be proactive and pursue what you want.

Although my options for the previous summer were limited due to the pending surgery, I managed to shadow a great mentor who was a successful real estate agent in Clarksville. The uncertainty of the pandemic led me to put off thoughts of graduate school and pursue this route. I became a licensed realtor in my hometown, but after four months in, I knew I didn't like it and wanted to quit. I spent the next two years doing a job I was miserable at, thinking it would get better, and ignoring my gut feeling to quit and move on. My health paid the price.

A combination of stress, loneliness, and outright discouragement put me in a miserable slump. Ending my life became a constant thought, and I wrote many suicide notes at my office desk, insisting to myself that today would be it.

A host of physical health problems emerged in 2022, beginning with dreadful back pain that reached the point where I could barely dress myself. This persisted for virtually the entire year, and despite appointments with several doctors, the true cause was never detected. A year off the weights, plus stretching and physical therapy, helped get my body in working order again. Then there was a series of nasal and congestion problems that lasted for months, making it difficult to breathe and sleep through the night. My Crohn's was also aggravated again, and a painful spell overtook me in the fall. I was sick as a dog, and my GI doctor loaded me up on more pills. I don't think the pills ever helped.

Again, it seemed that I just had to wait out this spell, which lasted a few months. Ironically, that year marked the beginning of my personal recovery, and it was desperately needed. I needed to focus on my health and get myself cured—once and for all.

During this time, I saw an allergy specialist who tested me for dozens of allergies, none of which I tested positive for. In January 2023, he asked out loud a question I had wondered for years: "Is the plan to stay on Remicade for life?" I'll forever be grateful to this allergist for having the courage to ask this question, and for giving me the confidence to do the same thing. I began researching alternative treatments to Crohn's disease, discovering Dr. Mark Hyman along the way, and listened to Dr. Hyman's interview with Dr. George Papanicolaou. In short, I went down the functional medicine rabbit hole. To hear two intelligent men—two doctors after all!—seriously speaking about alternatives to conventional medicine gave me tremendous hope and encouragement.

I knew I had to escape my current job and started looking for options. I didn't know what I wanted to do with my life; I still wasn't sure whether I wanted to live. At the time, my most recent happy memories were the fall of 2019, when I was healthy, doing well in school, and still had contact with my classmates. I thought about graduate school and how I could possibly reconstruct these circumstances, while also resetting my career and life goals. I loved economics as an undergraduate, so I began applying to graduate programs.

In what can only be considered a quintessential God thing, I was offered a scholarship to Troy University in Alabama.

It felt good to try something new, but I almost instantly regretted it. I knew nobody at Troy and was the only one in two of my three classes. Having worked with people twice my age and older out of college, I realized I had gone almost three years without talking to my contemporaries. You'll be bad at anything after a three-year hiatus, and I felt like a square peg in a round hole when trying to relate to the students and people there. My Crohn's was still not in control, and symptoms continued to plague me during my first semester.

TAKING CONTROL

I suppose people have many reasons for attending graduate school. Most are probably there to advance their career or fulfill a requirement to land a certain job. These were my objectives as well. I wanted to parlay the degree into a job with a think tank or in academia. However, my primary objective was to finally overcome Crohn's—to put myself in a position where I could find a new doctor, read more about alternative healing protocols, and physically get away from Vanderbilt. Things had run their course with my doctors in Nashville. What I needed was time and a place where I could heal myself.

Throughout high school and college, I let Crohn's disease hold me back. When you are sick at eleven or twelve, and indoctrinated by your doctors to believe that you'll never live a normal life, it eventually gets fixed in your head. You believe what they tell you, and though your social life is expected to bloom in high school and college, you hold yourself back on the false premise that you can never leave your house for fear of not finding a bathroom. It also makes big life decisions difficult. For one, you get accustomed to a series of regular appointments and infusions. You feel you can never get far from home, go on vacation, take risks, go out, and just live because you have been taught for years to keep Crohn's top of mind. In short, it makes planning out your life very challenging. This is no way to live, and I had to get myself unstuck before it was too late.

As I dove deeper into seeking God's help to overcome Crohn's, I started to imagine a life without this disease. We grew up going to church. Yet for me, I never saw faith as playing a major role in overcoming Crohn's. Neither the doctors nor the hospital I went to encouraged nor dismissed the spiritual component to healing. They took a largely secular, scientific approach—as you would expect of conventional medicine. Still sick, and feeling almost forsaken by my doctors, I began a serious effort to look to God for help. He helped me gain a clear picture for the first time of what I wanted: to be healthy and finally alleviate Crohn's disease in order to live a truly abundant life. None of the career and family aspirations I envisioned were ever going to happen until I finally overcame Crohn's.

My symptoms were awful during the fall semester. I could rarely sit for more than ten or fifteen minutes before needing to use the bathroom. I fired Vanderbilt Hospital and started seeing a GI doctor in Ozark, Alabama. He was initially on board with my desire to taper off Remicade. However, after my second visit with him in the spring of 2024, a gut feeling told me not to trust him or ever come back. After I had been waiting over an hour, he came into the room and stayed for less than a minute. He refused to let me come off Remicade and suggested this move could cause cancer. I responded that Remicade itself can cause cancer. He didn't deny this. Before our extremely short appointment ended, he began talking about the need to schedule a colonoscopy. My mind was made up before he finished speaking: I was through with him and would cure myself.

With virtually nothing to lose, and obviously against all official medical advice, I went cold turkey and quit Remicade. I was going to trust my gut and take my chances with my own body. I was determined to heal myself naturally, or die trying. It was one of the best decisions I ever made.

Chapter Two

CROHN'S AND COLITIS, IBD AND IBS

"All disease begins in the gut."

—HIPPOCRATES

Crohn's and ulcerative colitis are the two most prevalent forms of inflammatory bowel disease (IBD). Broadly speaking, IBD is a lifelong gut disorder primarily characterized by inflammation in the gastrointestinal (GI) tract.[12] But the symptoms of IBD can manifest in other areas of the body, including external organs; it is not confined to the gut. One adage of Crohn's disease is that it can show up anywhere in the body, from the lips to the anus.

Crohn's and colitis, and IBD more broadly, are classified as autoimmune diseases. Autoimmune stands for *your* immune system—"auto" meaning "self" or "autonomous" along with your immune system. By definition, the immune system refers to the integrated system of organs, tissues, cells, and cell products that differentiate your body from foreign substances and is capable of neutralizing or harming these substances as needed. Its job is to protect you by identifying foreign threats, communicating with other cells in your body, and launching an attack against them —whether it's a cancer cell, a toxin, a parasite, or something you ate. The first line of defense for your immune system is your skin, but the immune system is spread throughout the body, including the digestive system. We've all heard of the importance of having a strong immune system. It is vital to keeping your body healthy and requires vigilance to maintain a high level of performance. Healthy eating and exercise have long been recognized as factors that keep the immune system healthy and reduce the risk of you getting sick.

The immune system is one of the best things about your body. But strangely, the immune system is sometimes responsible for making you sick. At least that's how it's taught or understood by conventional medicine. The culprit for Crohn's and colitis remains unknown officially, but they are believed to be caused by the immune system attacking itself and the body: The immune system becomes angry, and it quickly manifests very painfully by inflaming portions of the intestines. Here again is what differentiates the two diseases: It depends on where in the GI tract the inflammation shows up.

Between Crohn's and colitis, Crohn's disease is the most all-encompassing of the two. Ulcerative colitis affects the mucosal layer of the colon and rectum, while Crohn's can be found along the entire GI tract. The symptoms of IBD include stomach pain and bloating, nausea, vomiting, poor appetite, weight loss, weight gain, diarrhea, bloody stool, fistula, and hemorrhoids.

It never made sense to me that the body would attack itself, and if it truly did, finding out why would be the most important thing. The key to overall health may lie in keeping your immune system healthy. When you are sick, it's important to look deeply into the root causes of your disease. It's not necessarily that your body is attacking itself, but that your body is having a series of terrible reactions to external and internal factors. It could be the food you eat, what you drink, your environment, trauma, toxins, a poor mindset, a bad job, isolation, or a combination of all of these. Even some of the medical literature is starting to acknowledge this, with one publication writing, "Many environmental factors can potentially trigger IBD."[13]

I originally thought that Crohn's disease took its name simply from the word "chronic," meaning "lasting for a long period of time or marked by frequent recurrence." Conventional medicine teaches this—that the disease is with you forever. By this understanding, conventional medicine instills the belief that the best you can ever hope to do is manage your symptoms or achieve remission. The goal of this book is to teach you otherwise.

Crohn's disease actually takes its name from the doctor who is credited with "discovering" it in 1932, Dr. Burrill B. Crohn.[14] Crohn's was originally thought to be caused by intestinal tuberculosis, and Dr. Crohn and his colleagues could not identify the source of this disease that affected the ileum. The cause of Crohn's remains, according to official medical understanding, unknown. I should back up and provide a quick sketch of the GI tract. You are surely familiar with both the large and small intestines. The large intestines are referred to as your colon. The small intestines are divided into three sections: the duodenum, the jejunum, and the ileum. Crohn's affects the entire GI tract, especially the ileum in the small intestine. This is one of the reasons that Crohn's disease is sometimes called chronic ileitis.

Although the exact cause of IBD is unknown, studies have linked "the cause of IBD to a combination of multiple factors, including genetic susceptibility, immune response dysfunction, gut microbial dysbiosis, and environmental factors."[15] In other words, someone could be born healthy but possess a propensity to get Crohn's or colitis. It may be triggered by stress, something they ate, or environmental factors.

For many sufferers, the symptoms of Crohn's and colitis seem to appear out of nowhere. You may feel fine, and then you get sharp stomach pains after eating lunch one day. Maybe you notice your energy levels or appetite dwindling, but you dismiss it as normal or not a big deal. That's how it happened for me. There seems to be an assumption we all possess while young that our bodies will work no matter what. If any symptoms arise, they are just a deviation from your otherwise healthy life. As we'll see later, it's important to look deeper at yourself and your health. While nothing in your routine may have changed, closer examination often reveals the root causes of your illness.

Still, symptoms are starting to show up. Since they don't know where the symptoms come from, the default position among doctors has been to treat the symptoms by placing patients on any one of many pharmaceutical products approved to treat Crohn's or colitis. Patients are often bounced around from medication to medication. A medicine will be used until it "stops working." Then, it's on to the next product. The protocol could be summed up as follows: flare, treat, remission, repeat. The process is absurd when you really think about it.

By contrast, the functional medicine approach seeks to address the root causes and heal the patient—by looking at their unique needs and treating them as individuals and not deferring to whatever official science or medicine says on the matter.

STRIVE TO BE HEALED

According to Western medical doctors, Crohn's disease is incurable. Crohn's patients are inundated with this alleged fact. I was.

Even if you manage to conquer all of your symptoms, you are not considered cured by medical standards. Rather you are in remission. The word remission is used by doctors because it carries the implication that even though you are asymptomatic, you are still sick and must continue with your appointments and medications. It is a very autocratic attitude that these doctors have toward their patients, in insisting that they are still sick when they feel fine.

I hope to show you that remission is a completely flawed notion. You shouldn't strive to be symptom-free and still sick. If you are symptom-free, why do the doctors still want to classify you as being sick? Is it to keep you on the medical rosters and on the pharmaceutical racket? Why would someone who is asymptomatic continue to get treated for a disease they do not feel? If you have reached the point of being able to exercise and eat as you would like, do you need to continue the charade of being sick? You should strive to be healed. Healed means the wound has been restored to health or soundness and requires no further attention from medical experts.

One of the first steps to healing yourself is a correct diagnosis. For example, irritable bowel syndrome (IBS) is a lesser form of IBD, not as severe (officially) as Crohn's and colitis—although you should talk to some of the people who have it. Some have theorized that there is only Crohn's disease, and that these other conditions all lead to Crohn's. In other words, there is a continuum, and Crohn's disease is at the far end on the most severe side. Some patients are initially diagnosed with IBS, then they get "upgraded" to ulcerative colitis, before they are finally declared a Crohn's patient by their GI doctor. This is worth keeping in mind, as treating one of these conditions is basically like treating them all. But it's also worth remembering that no case is identical. Crohn's may affect you differently than it did me. Similarly, ulcerative colitis may cause symptoms for one person that other UC patients don't experience. Each solution is tailored to your own unique needs and symptoms.

I don't want to come across as a cheerleader for Crohn's, but I want people to be diagnosed properly. It's possible that you could be misdiagnosed and that symptoms could appear in other areas that are dismissed by your doctor. Therefore, it is important to treat all of your symptoms, not just the area your physician identifies as sick or inflamed. Otherwise, you will never be fully healed. Your health may evolve as you get older and face new circumstances. For instance, say you get diagnosed with IBS at twenty. A few years later, as you are exposed to more stress, a new environment, and harmful toxins and chemicals, your diagnosis is upgraded to Crohn's.

During my first major episode of digestive tract troubles, I was never officially diagnosed with anything. Why? Part of it is the mystery of the body. Inflammation can come and go quickly, as can other symptoms. Doctors may perform blood tests and other procedures to identify the cause of these symptoms. But sometimes, your body does not give them a reason to diagnose—this can be so frustrating because you are in pain!

When I began seeking alternative treatments, I came across Jini Patel Thompson's work. She introduced the concept that all these conditions lead to Crohn's in the end and notes that it could be possible for someone's symptoms to slowly manifest into Crohn's. Each step along the way to this ultimate diagnosis reflects your body's present state of health. Initially, inflammation may have appeared in the colon, which would generally merit an ulcerative colitis diagnosis. Later, inflammation showed up in the ileum of the small intestine, which is more in line with Crohn's. The initial symptoms may have been triggered by a host of factors. Either not treated, or exacerbated by some new factor, the disease showed up in another portion of the GI tract.

RISK FACTORS

Historically, Crohn's disease has been more prevalent in the Western world, with fewer cases found in Africa, Asia, and South America. It is not groundbreaking to suggest that this is owed to the fact that people in the Western world tend to eat a modern Western diet—high in refined grains and sugar, very unlike other parts of the world where traditional diets and lifestyles prevail. But cases are beginning to rise in places where the disease was once not as common. For instance, there has been a yearly escalation of Crohn's diagnosis in Brazil since 1990.[16]

We are also told that Crohn's disease likely has a genetic component since cases tend to cluster in certain families. That may be true. One study reports that genetic heritability can be found in up to 12 percent of Crohn's patients.[17] IBD has been most common among children and adults in Western countries and among certain ethnic groups, such as the Ashkenazi Jews.[18]

However, an increasing amount of medical and scientific research is pointing to environmental and lifestyle factors as being contributors to IBD, Crohn's, and colitis, which makes sense. Certain families tend to have the same diet and lifestyle as one another, thus leading to more cases. If an urban family consumes a highly processed diet and multiple members of the family are diagnosed with Crohn's disease or IBD, can we conclude that genetics play a role? Maybe. But what about the family that lives in the country, grows their own food, and none of its members are diagnosed with any autoimmune conditions? Could we conclude that "good" genetics are to thank? Perhaps.

But the only clear distinction is the diet and lifestyle differences between the two families.

A 2019 article published in *Gastroenterology* reported that there are conditions of childhood that decrease one's risk of developing IBD. Lifestyle factors such as living near farm animals, having pets, and having two or more siblings all played a protective role against Crohn's disease. Living near farm animals, access to a personal toilet, having pets, and access to hot water were protective against ulcerative colitis. Physical activity was found to help prevent Crohn's, and so was breastfeeding. In fact, longer exposure to breastfeeding was associated with a decreased risk for the baby.[19]

In short, living the way many people did in an earlier America appears to generally keep your gut healthier. Factors such as natural birth, breastfeeding, multiple siblings, and living around livestock are all factors that decrease your likelihood of having Crohn's, or (most likely) getting sick in general.

On the flipside, other factors have been found to be associated with an increased likelihood of developing IBD. Cesarean birth was associated with Crohn's disease, as were surgeries such as appendectomy and tonsillectomy.[20] While a lack of breastfeeding is not an explicit risk factor for developing Crohn's or colitis, the authors added that "The absence of breastfeeding has been associated with colonization by *Clostridium difficile* [*C. diff*] and immune-mediated disease."[21] *C. diff* is a bacterium that can cause severe inflammation of the colon. Many of the ensuing symptoms are very similar to what you experience with Crohn's, including severe diarrhea, stomach pain, dehydration, and fever. During my 2011 hospitalization, I also contracted *C. diff*. (This meant remaining quarantined in addition to dealing with a Crohn's flare.)

This same article in *Gastroenterology* explained that smoking, urban living, antibiotic exposure, oral contraceptive use, consumption of soft drinks, and vitamin D deficiency were all found to increase the risk of developing IBD.[22] Antibiotics can alter the composition of your gut microbiome, increasing your risk of gastrointestinal problems.

INFLAMMATION

At the heart of Crohn's disease is inflammation. You may have heard the term, especially as there is more widespread awareness of Americans getting chronically sick. Without getting too into the weeds, here's the rundown on inflammation. According to the *Standard American Dictionary*, to inflame means to make more violent or intensify. Inflammation in the body is a localized protective reaction of tissue to irritation, injury, or infection, characterized by heat, redness, swelling, and pain. The goal of inflammation, or short-term acute inflammation, is to repair injury and promote healing. As we see with Crohn's and other autoimmune diseases, the problem is when inflammation becomes chronic.

Crohn's patients often suffer from severe inflammation of the small or large intestine, sometimes both. Picture your body getting angry on the inside. Your intestines swell, making it difficult for food to pass through. A healthy intestine is pink and pristine, round and open, allowing for the easy flow of food through the digestive system. This process becomes interrupted during a Crohn's flare, or a severe episode of colitis or IBD. Your intestines, and the entire GI tract, have basically ceased to function.

Conventional medicine resorts to dangerous pharmaceuticals, including biologics, that act as immunosuppressants. This essentially shuts down your immune system, blocking the way it was intended to function. You are left vulnerable to the flu, seasonal allergies, sinus infections, and other viruses, but *at least* your stomach is "healed." Even if this were true, it does not make sense to compromise the health of the rest of your body at the expense of healing one part.

The logic with this conventional approach is beyond flawed. You are not healed even after taking these drugs. To be healed means to restore to health or soundness, to cure. The best pharmaceutical products can do is mask the problem. They can temporarily cover them up, but they can never address the underlying issues, least of all cure you. When symptoms finally do subside with Crohn's disease, the period you enter into is called remission. Remission is not the same as being cured; rather, it is the lessening of intensity. The symptoms and underlying causes remain, you just don't feel or notice them under the remission phase.

The question about inflammation is, why? Your body is self-interested in so many ways. Your stomach growls when you're hungry. Your throat becomes parched when you're thirsty. Your eyelids become heavy when you're sleepy. You sweat to cool off. Soreness after an intense workout signals that your muscles need a break. In short, your body has so many incredible signals that instinctively alert you to meet its needs. This background makes it all the more important to understand why the immune system would attack the gastrointestinal tract in your body. Why do the intestines suddenly become inflamed and start to reject food, your body's fuel? Why do the bowels cease to function, or start to empty so frequently that you can seldom do anything else but anticipate your next trip to the bathroom? It sounds crazy, but that's how Crohn's disease is simplified to most patients: *Your body is attacking itself, so take these man-made drugs to shut it down.*

It's possible that the symptoms are instead an adverse reaction to certain foods, chemicals, toxins, environmental factors, or traumatic experiences. Your body may be acting in self-interest or in self-defense, but the manifestation is extremely painful and harmful to your overall health. It's like the legend of the Dutch farmer who burned his barn to rid it of rats. The rats were gone, but so was the barn.

Luckily, you don't have to rid your body of rats, but there are metaphorical rats you need to rid your body, home, and environment of. Here, we come to the functional medicine approach. It's the approach of treating your body as an integrated system, while also bearing in mind that you were uniquely created and have your own nuances that cause your body to function and react in ways others won't.

GOING DRUG-FREE

After I fired my conventional doctors and decided to heal myself, my first decision was to get off the drugs I'd been taking.

Gone were the biologics. Gone was the irritating need to schedule an appointment and drive an hour to an infusion center every six weeks. Instead, I joined a new gym that had a sauna. I spent several hours there over the course of two weeks. Sweating is one of the best ways to detox your body, and I wanted to get the last remnants of Remicade out of my system.

It would be a bit generous to say I was off all medicine. I started appointments with a functional medicine provider in Texas named Dr. Ross. He introduced me to probiotics, in addition to natural anti-inflammatories such as fish oil. A combination of these supplements and following his recommended low-FODMAP (fermentable oligosaccharides, disaccharides, monosaccharides, and polyols) diet (more in Chapter 6) really improved my condition. After the supplements were implemented, I went on a remarkable ten-day to two-week stretch with zero symptoms. I felt completely healthy and born-again in the health sense. But after this initial success, symptoms reappeared, and his next recommendation was the elemental diet drink.

The elemental diet drink is a delicious meal replacement supplement that is very easy on your stomach and entire GI tract. I would recommend it to anyone, sick or not, just to give your body a break from solid food, as your digestive tract does need a rest now and then. A later chapter on nutrition will explain its benefits in greater detail. There are so many nuances to becoming drug-free, but it has been the most liberating experience of my life. I have never felt so good, and I want everyone with IBD, Crohn's, or colitis to enjoy this amazing gift.

If you are trying to overcome Crohn's, or any autoimmune disease, it is important to keep in mind that there is no "one size fits all" solution. In fact, there are still aspects I struggle with from time to time, and it requires constant vigilance on multiple fronts, including nutrition, fitness, and spiritual well-being. Your journey to becoming drug-free may look different from mine, and that's okay. My goal is to provide you with the inspiration and a basic template to get started.

It is important to take inventory of your life and take a deep look back at the time you were diagnosed, and recognize what may have initially triggered your symptoms. Equally important is to identify the times in your life when you have felt your best. You will be able to see patterns during your down times, days when you were really struggling with symptoms, and the times when you felt great/symptom-free, healthy, and fit as a fiddle.

When it comes to examining the root causes of your health problems, you must reconcile with what went wrong, accept that you cannot change it, and resolve to live a healthy and abundant life going forward. Even if you are not diagnosed with anything, or have no condition to overcome, I highly recommend keeping a food and exercise diary, which is a step I'll flesh out in a later chapter. I have now been drug-free for over a year, and I'm truly healthier, happier, and fitter than I've ever been.

A CALL TO ACTION

Why does IBD matter? One recent academic paper said that between 1990 and 2019, there was a 47 percent increase in the incidence of IBD globally, with a 69 percent rise in mortality from IBD worldwide during the same time period.[23] That fact alone makes this topic worth exploring. A lifelong disease on the rise calls for action, especially given the harmful effects the disease can have on those who live with it. It's even more alarming when considering the increase in cases among children. According to one case report, pediatric Crohn's disease was up 148 percent between 2007 and 2016.[24]

Those with Crohn's or colitis are six times more likely to develop colon cancer than the general population.[25] There is also an enormous financial cost to these diseases for the patients personally and the healthcare system. According to one scholarly journal article on Crohn's, "Patients with IBD also have higher rates of depression and anxiety than the general population."[26] Your mood and mental well-being are intrinsically linked to what happens inside your gut. Your gut is sometimes referred to as your second brain. The connection is real, and imbalances in the gastrointestinal tract can manifest throughout the rest of the body, including a poor mental state.

Those with IBD and other autoimmune conditions carry an awful stigma that they are sick for life. This is especially harmful for children to hear, but this is an aspect of Crohn's and autoimmune diseases that needs to be disproven, and those who have naturally cured themselves have a responsibility to show others how it can be done. The phrase "sick for life" creates a self-fulfilling prophecy for many patients. They may genuinely feel fine on days after their diagnosis. But because of the dogma, they have internalized the belief that no matter how well they feel, they are still sick. It's no way to live, and it's a terrible idea to instill into boys and young men. Men are supposed to take risks and take an intentional approach to life. But there is a dreadful trap that men who are diagnosed with these problems can fall into. Tethered to routine appointments and medications, there is a tendency to play life safe and become risk-averse. This is contrary to our nature and leaves unfulfilled potential on the table of your life story.

An often-overlooked effect of IBD and autoimmune disease is the poor quality of life that can accompany them. The embarrassing nature of GI symptoms can easily affect your personal life and strain relationships. Those with Crohn's and colitis are warned to always have a bathroom handy, in addition to the constant need to be mindful of what they eat and drink. One bite of the wrong food may send you to the bathroom for the remainder of a party or social gathering. There are missed school days due to appointments, and the challenge of trying to make it through school and work while dealing with symptoms. In many ways, Crohn's and autoimmune disease can hold you back personally and professionally. With the need to factor in appointments, medications, symptoms, and the general unknowns of Crohn's, it makes career decisions and other major life choices all the more difficult to plan and pursue. A person cannot truly live as their happiest, healthiest, wealthiest, and most productive version of themselves with the stigma and insecurity that can accompany autoimmune disease. Thankfully for you and so many others, there is an alternative.

Chapter Three

THE PROBLEM WITH MODERN HEALTHCARE

"Semmelweis Reflex: A human behavioral tendency to stick to preexisting beliefs and to reject fresh ideas that contradict them."
—VIPIN GUPTA, *WORLD NEUROSURGERY*

Anyone who has visited an American hospital, doctor's office, or clinic is acutely aware of the many operational problems our healthcare facilities face. Lengthy wait times, inefficient staffing, inadequate care, and questionable provider competency are just a few of the issues commonly faced by anyone who needs medical services.

Upon entering any hospital, doctor's office, or walk-in clinic, the first question almost always asked by the desk attendant is not "what's wrong with you?" but rather "what insurance do you have?" Your co-pay, a copy of your insurance card, and a photo ID must be presented, and forms that ask questions such as "Do you feel safe at home?" must be completed before addressing why you showed up in the first place. Imagine walking into a grocery store and being questioned immediately by the store manager about how you are going to pay for the food and other items you place in your buggy. "Cash or card?" You would leave. Yet, in its current state, our medical system operates on a similar basis.

Instinctively, I am the type of person who avoids going to the doctor at all costs, which makes my experience with Crohn's all the more ironic. Yet it is true: Only when things got extremely bad did my family ever turn to the hospital. Although going to the hospital became routine, I never liked it. There is an unhealthy mental element to going to the doctor and hospital frequently as a child and teenager. Not that Vanderbilt and other hospitals are gory, but it's not where children are supposed to be. We're supposed to be outside and in school. I know the feeling of wasting precious time in my adolescence on appointments that ultimately did little or no good. Even then, I was starting to develop a feeling that I needed to end this dead-end cycle. With Crohn's and colitis, there is usually the dreaded blood test that gets ordered immediately following your visit. This only adds to the time you spend in the hospital and means another needle. It's a frustrating routine.

Before quitting Vanderbilt, I played a little game with my doctor's office and staff each time—although I was the only player and the only one who noticed, apparently. Before each visit, they gave me a tablet with nearly a hundred questions to answer before I could see the doctor. The answers were always for *your* health so we can better understand *your* unique needs and care for *you* better. With each question, there was always a "good" answer and a "bad" answer. For example, "How do you feel?" would be answered with "excellent" for the good answer and "terrible" for the bad answer.

No matter how I answered the questions (which were the same each time), I was never asked about my responses. For convenience, I simply selected all of the "good" answers, expecting to hear a "Wow, you must be doing great!" I heard nothing at all. On the next visit, I selected all of the "bad" answers—which, if true, would mean I was either dead or so bad off that there is no way I could have shown up for my appointment. After selecting the "bad" answers, I got no reaction from my doctor or the staff and quickly deduced that the entire process was some insurance requirement, hospital procedure, or federal mandate that required this ridiculous series of questions before I could see the doctor or nurse practitioner. People respond to incentives, and once I realized there was no difference in the care I received regardless of how I responded, I took it completely unseriously. This is just one of many examples of how bureaucracy harms healthcare outcomes.

For almost all parties involved, the healthcare system in America is screwed up. And the screw ups are not just procedural and administrative. Whenever my doctor or nurse practitioner finally came to the room, it was—without fail—the same old, same old. Rarely was anything new or meaningful about my health discussed. Many times, I would inform them of symptoms I had experienced that had resolved before my appointment. In which case, my doctor could only offer a response like, "Well, let us know in six months if you have the same symptoms or any issues."

THE MEDICAL INDUSTRY

There are numerous flaws with the testing, reasoning, and assertions made within the medical industry, especially the medicines used to treat Crohn's disease.

I am not necessarily anti-doctor. People have practiced medicine for thousands of years. Physicians are part of our civilization, and can be a great source of understanding. That being said, doctors are not above criticism when called for, and it is fair to question their practices at times—just as every other profession deserves criticism when appropriate. There are some good doctors, no doubt. But until doctors curtail some of the absurd practices they follow, I believe it's best to trust your own intuition and remain healthy on your own. Among her many wise sayings, my grandmother could never emphasize enough that medicine was still a *practice*—and we ought to approach doctors with this in mind.

One of the most persistent myths surrounding our healthcare system is that doctors are owed our unquestioning devotion, and their wisdom need not be questioned. If they prescribe a medicine, take it. If they tell you not to do something, obey. If they tell you not to eat something, follow through. There is a remarkable lack of personalization that accompanies a visit to the doctor's office. Gone are the days of the "family doctor" where the doc took his time and got to know the person. In its place is a commercialized approach to medicine that treats every patient the same, regardless of medical and family history and their unique health challenges. For too long, I blindly followed the advice and instructions of my doctors. There were times when I felt fine, but other times when I still struggled with the same symptoms. I was never cured while in their care.

In the modern era, hospitals and doctors' offices possess an aura that instantly conveys the supposed intelligence and expertise of those working inside. There is no question that it requires a great deal of talent and academic fortitude to survive the rigors of medical school, yet there is increasing reason to doubt that those who graduate from these institutions are truly qualified. Heather Mac Donald of the Manhattan Institute has highlighted how hospitals, medical schools, and medical associations, in their admissions and hiring decisions, are prioritizing characteristics such as race as opposed to test scores and intelligence—leading some of the smartest students to say, "Now that I see what is happening in medicine, I will do something else."[27]

Credentialism in the American economy has created the illusion of omniscience in many professions, including medicine. However, we should never give our blind loyalty to any profession, especially if they are trying to induce you to do something you instinctively know is wrong or harmful. You wouldn't hire a lawyer who is constantly urging you to divorce your spouse, or hire a roofer who is adamant your shingles are worn out. There is an adage about never asking a barber if you need a haircut, because the answer is always yes. These people may not be deceitful, but they are ultimately acting out of self-interest by creating more business opportunities by any means necessary. The body is a complex integrated system. As much as we know, there is still so much we don't know about ourselves. This is where the arrogance and omniscience of doctors always bothered me. They probably know very little about their own body and health, yet are adamant they know what's wrong with you and how to cure or treat you.

Unfortunately, the healthcare industry relies on a lot of people getting sick and staying sick. In fact, healthcare is sometimes referred to as sick care, for the goal is not to truly cure you. This is an instinctive point for anyone who has ever visited the hospital. You rarely get just one appointment. There are always follow-up visits, and patients are routinely referred to other providers when the one they are paying to see cannot heal them.

Again, conventional doctors attempt to *treat* symptoms, not heal symptoms and address the underlying causes. In other words, as long as you stay attached to your conventional treatment plan, you are never going to be fully well. It's my goal to help you seek healing elsewhere.

SPECIALIZATION

Throughout human history, almost every society has had the majority of its population engaged in growing or finding food. Indeed, in the early years of the newly formed United States, some 90 percent of the population was employed in agriculture. Today, only 1 percent of Americans farm.[28] The Industrial Revolution made energy cheaper and machines more efficient, and gradually people were able to move from farm life into other ventures. We have become specialized.

Americans now enjoy a host of products that would not exist if most people still tilled the land. We enjoy washing machines, cars, airplanes, computers, and numerous other things because people are now freed up to make and provide these goods and services. The problem is that as we have become increasingly specialized, we have become increasingly disconnected from our food source. With fewer watchful eyes tending to our food supply, growers and governments have allowed increasingly harmful substances to be applied to the food we eat. This is making us sick and decreasing our life span.

This has been an especially harmful process for men. Men have shifted into more sedentary jobs that often require hours of screentime. It's not a healthy development and counter to how we are wired to live.

Specialization has also occurred in the medical field. Medical schools have subdivided the human body. Today, doctors may know more than ever about specific parts, yet understand less about the body as a whole. No doubt this specialization has led to great discoveries about certain body parts, but it is a dreadful way to approach most patients, especially those with IBD whose symptoms can show up in so many areas. If the body is just a bunch of parts, then they can be fixed individually, and you can be made well. For those with IBD, it is vitally important to treat the body like the complex integrated system that it is—with no one-size-fits-all solution. What works for me may not work for you, and vice versa.

MEDICAL MYTHS

For centuries, doctors recognized the importance of preventative care—ensuring that patients stayed physically active and ate a proper diet. It was not understood precisely how everything worked, but there was an inherent understanding that the body was a complex, integrated system.

As we'll see in Chapter 6, eating healthy is the preeminent aspect of preventing disease and illness, yet most doctors completely neglect the role of nutrition. They may, of course, throw a bone at the fitness gurus by recommending you *eat right* without ever going into detail about what this means. But a lot of medical literature, including journal articles and reviews, still dismisses the prospect of using food and nutrition as medicine. For example, one article from *Therapeutic Advances in Gastro-enterology* stated that "there are currently no data to suggest that these approaches [dietary modifications] have any role in the induction or maintenance of remission."[29] This is the typical sentiment expressed by mainstream doctors and hospitals: *Food hasn't been studied, so we don't know if it works.* Following up on this dismissive predisposition is usually the instruction that since food hasn't been proven, it's best not to even try to use food and natural protocols to fix yourself. My own intuition said to "go for it" and ignore the advice of Big Doctor.

Largely due to lack of funding and disinterest from the powers that be, "there is insufficient scientific support to give health care providers more options regarding dietary therapies."[30] But even if doctors aren't, the public is hungry for more information on how food and autoimmune diseases are connected. Over the last twenty-three years, there has been steady growth in the number of documents related to nutrition and Crohn's disease—reflecting growing public interest in the prospect of using food to treat yourself.[31]

Based on my experience, here are a few common understandings about modern-day doctors, hospitals, and medicines that need to be rethought.

MYTH: EVERYONE SHOULD HAVE A PRIMARY CARE DOCTOR

Regular checkups imply that something is consistently wrong. If nothing is wrong, why go to the doctor? That is, why are patients attending a scheduled appointment just to confirm that nothing is wrong?

This is not to discourage those with an active condition or injury from maintaining regular appointments until they are healed. But on the whole, you are typically the best judge of how you are doing. Weigh yourself daily. Take a look in the mirror. Do you look fit or fat? Are you happy or distressed? Have you exercised today? In short, have some common sense when it comes to your well-being. If you feel great, have a positive mindset, and are exercising and eating right, I see no need to pay a doctor to confirm what you already know to be true.

In my experience, typical medical doctors treat patients from either one of two extremes: They are either remarkably indifferent and dismiss whatever symptoms you are experiencing, or they take the hypochondriac approach. When they act on the latter, they instantly want labs and other tests done, and may rush in a prescription for you. I've been on both ends of this. For months leading up to my initial hospitalization, my symptoms were largely ignored and thought to be just common childhood stomach aches. Anecdotally, you may be aware of stories in which patients showed up at a hospital or doctor's office, sensing that they possessed a burning affliction, and, tragically, they were either dismissed or ignored and died a short time later. Likewise, how many people have shown up to the doctor with minor ailments (or no ailments at all), yet either under the mistaken guise of helping the patient—or perhaps with more sinister intentions—an entirely unnecessary surgery was performed or medication given?

To be sure, I am more than grateful that doctors can easily cure strep throat—a common childhood ailment that, along with pneumonia, contributed to the death of all-American Notre Dame football star George Gipp in 1920.[32] And we are also glad medicine can easily treat scabs, bruises, and minor injuries such as a blister—which killed President Calvin Coolidge's son in 1924.[33] These unfortunate incidents were the result of medical ignorance in certain respects, but the America of today has a greater understanding of how to treat such occurrences.

My long-standing belief is that doctors should be for emergencies only: delivering babies, addressing gunshot wounds, healing broken legs, etc. In many cases, most medical problems you have can be addressed by a nurse or nurse practitioner. If you were bleeding and had to choose, would you rather see a nurse or a doctor anyway? You are allowed to "walk-off" some injuries, and soap and water will prevent infection of a lot of minor wounds.

Trust your gut, and use doctors on an as-needed basis.

MYTH: YOU NEED THIS TEST

So many times, I have blindly followed the doctor's orders to have a certain test or procedure done. I had no choice in most cases. Those with IBD or IBS are likely used to the annual or biennial colonoscopy ritual. These tests are conducted while the patient is well, and the GI doctor is searching for signs of illness. But if the patient is not sick, no symptoms may appear. So, what is the point of the test? When you consider that symptoms could show up the next day after the test has been performed, it makes no sense to perform routine tests on a healthy person.

A colonoscopy is the test most associated with middle age and IBD. Crohn's and IBD patients typically have this procedure done once every two years. In my experience, almost every colonoscopy I had just confirmed what I already knew—that I felt fine. However, I was always very uncomfortable with the stuff they injected into my IV and the pills they gave me beforehand. I have no idea what it was or what it was for, and I regret blindly taking these. Before my last colonoscopy, I vividly remember having to sign a form authorizing my doctor to administer a blood transfusion in the event of an emergency. Of course I signed, like any obedient patient would. But the whole time I was thinking, *if they can screw up a colonoscopy to the point where I need a blood transfusion to survive this, I'm not sure I want to live to see the results.*

They do colonoscopies in Europe and have problems there as well. A major study conducted out of northern Europe found that the procedure doesn't save as many lives as doctors and researchers once believed. Moreover, colonoscopies are not without risk, including major bleeding, perforation, and infection.[34] That's something they don't tell you—these tubes are used over and over!

Regardless, inflammation can come and go so quickly that a brief scan or scope of your colon is likely to reveal very little meaningful information. Moreover, the medical community pushes colonoscopies, as well as cancer screening and other tests—generally marked as an annual or coming-of-age event. Any industry is going to lobby for more business, why would the medical industry be any different?

I use my intuition. Colonoscopies always either confirmed what I already knew—either that I felt fine, or felt like I was on death's door (which happened only once). Additionally, I had one of these tests performed just months before my last flare, and it showed "all-clear" throughout my intestinal tract. Inflammation can set in quickly, and a colonoscopy failed to give any indication that a flare-up was one the way. Use your own judgment in the same manner when determining whether or not to get a test.

MRIs and CAT scans are also common tests run on Crohn's patients. While MRIs are generally regarded as safe, CAT scans expose the body to radiation. Regardless, it has become my belief that medical tests should be avoided at all costs. For most people, they are never needed. The trouble with Crohn's disease, colitis, and IBD is that these tests become routine.

This is an aside, but it's not just tests for IBS or IBD that need rethinking. Women are practically required to get a mammogram to screen for breast cancer. If women are asymptomatic, and in good health, it's fair to question whether these tests are really necessary. Again, testing for cancer, illness, or any medical condition may be a modern miracle, but the entire premise rests on the philosophy of treating sick patients—rather than preventing them from getting sick altogether. We know, for instance, that the Inuit peoples of the Arctic were among the last indigenous groups on earth to transition to a modern diet high in sugar, white flour, and chemicals. After the 1970s-era culinary transformation, breast cancer became a common occurrence among Inuit women. Consider this: Early Arctic explorer Vilhjalmur Stefansson cited the findings of Captain

George B. Leavitt, who found only one case of cancer in nearly fifty years among the natives.[35] Is the lesson that women need a mammogram, or that women should try to avoid white flour and sugar? Pink T-shirts may raise awareness of breast cancer, but changing your diet and lifestyle might prevent it altogether.

We need a more proactive approach and a return to preventative care, rather than the current system that focuses on treating illness, often a condition that never would have developed if people and their physicians prioritized a consistent, healthy lifestyle from an early age.

MYTH: FITNESS IS PRESCRIBED

There is a complete lack of emphasis placed by modern doctors on the importance of exercise and healthy living. I have witnessed so many overweight people at hospitals and doctors' offices over the years, often seeking treatment for an ailment or illness, such as a bad ankle or diabetes, that might have been prevented altogether if they had followed a healthy exercise and diet regimen, instead of being prescribed pharmaceuticals. This is one of the most intuitive aspects of health that professionals miss, leaving room to wonder if its absence is intentional. Moreover, the neglect of exercise and fitness in modern medical facilities runs counter to physicians' advice to patients for thousands of years.

The connection between exercise and health was long understood, and widespread even, among physicians in the late 1800s and early 1900s. In fact, the term "physical education" began to appear in American medical literature before the Civil War. Dr. John Warren of Harvard University published *Physical Education and the Preservation of Health* in 1846. He noted "that health may be preserved to a late period of life by the use of those things, which are friendly, and the avoidance of those which are noxious. Most diseases are the consequences of violations of the laws of nature, sometimes the result of ignorance, more frequently of inattention."[36]

But as scientific and technological innovation gave rise to new medical tools, such as X-rays and better surgical equipment, there was almost certainly an urge to use them. This contributed to the "treatment" approach to health rather than the traditional approach of prevention altogether.

Jack Berryman, in "Exercise Is Medicine: A Historical Perspective," writes, "Bacteriology and the new germ theory impacted past beliefs about public health, disease, and infections, new surgical techniques put more emphasis on treating than preventing, new drugs could now cure, and x-rays along with other instruments moved diagnosis beyond previous limit."[37]

The American Medical Association gained more power and control over the education of physicians in the early 1900s, and a greater emphasis was placed on "cure rather than prevention." It was also at this time that physicians began to specialize—a harmful trend, as mentioned earlier.

Berryman adds, "exercise began to lose the attention previously displayed by many physicians."[38] This is another intuitive point, and surely you have witnessed it yourself. How many times has a walk outdoors or an hour in the gym made you feel ten times better? Unfortunately, there are so many fat people sitting in waiting rooms at the doctor's office, when the answer is so obvious—stand up and go for a walk outside!

A later chapter is devoted to the role of exercise and movement, but for now, don't let yourself miss out on this most obvious and enjoyable aspect of health.

MYTH: SURGERY IS THE SOLUTION

Irreversible surgery is a tragic reality for many Crohn's and IBD patients. Although I had a stricture removed and a resection performed, I would not recommend it to other patients. There's no use dwelling on water over the dam. I'm grateful my surgeon did a good job and that I made a quick recovery. If I were advising patients, I would strongly suggest an alternative treatment, such as an all-liquid elemental diet for a few months, to allow your intestines to heal.

Here are a few problems with the surgical option. For one, the disease is supposedly incurable. The same people operating on you will only reinforce this notion. Even after you have a section of your intestines removed, the disease is still there and can spread to the other areas each time you have a portion removed. Too many IBD patients have not had just one surgery on their bowel, but multiple. It makes my stomach hurt to think about having your intestines removed, piece by piece, over multiple surgeries.

Also, surgery is never without risk. One study of 103 Crohn's patients at the largest hospital in Latin America found that "32% had postoperative complications."[39] These problems arose within thirty days of surgery. Of twenty-seven surgical complications, fourteen were related to the abdominal wound itself, while thirteen were related to infection. Meanwhile, six patients had clinical complications, including postoperative ileus, pneumonia, and deep venous thrombosis.[40] The paper adds that "stoma creation was associated with increased risk for complications."[41]

An academic paper published in *Nutrients* noted that another consequence of surgery was that "subjects who undergo extensive bowel resection have an increased risk of vitamin B12 malabsorption."[42] The paper added that a stricture—the scarring of your intestine—is a common occurrence, affecting about 70 percent of Crohn's patients. Most of these patients require surgery within the first twenty years of their diagnosis. However, "post-operative complications are common in patients undergoing intestinal resection, with a risk rate of 30% in the pre-biologic era."[43]

Can you imagine having an incurable disease, knowing that surgery in twenty years' time is allegedly inevitable? My primary concern before my surgery was how the removal of twelve to eighteen inches of small intestine would affect my absorption capacity. I was told it wouldn't. But the primary job of the small intestine, including the ileum, is to absorb nutrients. Subtracting workspace for absorption to occur will certainly adversely affect this capacity. Lastly, it can't be stressed enough that this is an irreversible procedure. You only have one body. Do you really want to surrender any of your vital organs in the hope that you might feel better after the fact? The human body is remarkably capable of healing itself, even if the process can be long and frustrating. Bet on yourself, and not the surgeons. Treat yourself naturally.

MEDICATIONS ARE NOT CURES

My generation has grown up inundated with television commercials for pharmaceutical products. A significant portion of television advertising comes from pharmaceutical companies. Now, advertising for certain types of foods or vacation destinations makes sense, because viewers can decide for themselves whether they want to buy that brand of chips or take a trip there. Advertising directly to consumers for pharmaceuticals always struck me as odd and bothersome. For one, viewers cannot prescribe themselves the medicines they see ads for. Secondly, in a two-minute commercial, at least ninety seconds is devoted to a narrator in the background telling you all of the side effects. It can be fun to mock some of the serious side effects of medications designed to treat trivial medical conditions. If you have an occasional cough or itchy elbow, you're probably not really willing to risk cancer or suicide to make it go away.

One thing that stands out immediately about all of the IBD and IBS medications is the disclaimer that this is not a cure, but rather a tool to help manage symptoms. When Remicade was approved for children, Steven Galson, MD, director of the FDA's Center for Drug Evaluation and Research, said, "Remicade is not a cure."[44] The goal of these medications is only to treat and mask symptoms, without getting to the root cause of why you got sick in the first place. A lot of the side effects caused by these medicines are identical to the symptoms you experience with autoimmune disease in the first place. If diarrhea is a common symptom of IBD and IBS, how are you to discern whether the diarrhea you subsequently experience is caused by your IBD/IBS or by the medication taken to treat your condition? Are common side effects somehow better if they result from medication rather than from your body's troubled state?

In the United States, the Food and Drug Administration holds the keys to allowing new prescription drugs on the market to treat virtually any condition. It's well worth examining this agency, and how it determines whether or not a drug should be approved.

"Regulatory captures" refers to the economic phenomenon in government-agency-business relations in which departments created by the federal government to oversee private enterprises—to ensure they are not harming consumers—become in effect captured or hostage to the very businesses they are supposed to regulate. If you are an executive within a federal agency, and can be promised a high-paying job in the private sector, why would you take action to harm that industry?

The FDA is not immune to this corruption mechanism. Indeed, a host of former directors have gone on to work for pharmaceutical companies. From 1981 to 2019, the US had ten FDA commissioners. All but one took a job with a pharmaceutical company following the end of their tenure or resignation.[45] The full scale of corruption is beyond the scope of this book, but the agency responsible for the medications you consume is not without its own problems.

Moreover, few likely take the time to read the official studies, reports, and statements produced by the FDA on any of the medications it approves, including those for Crohn's, such as infliximab (Remicade), prednisone, upadacitinib (Rinvoq), and adalimumab (Humira).

Remicade is just one example of many drugs prescribed for Crohn's disease, but it demonstrates all the issues with medication as a treatment. Remicade is a biologic drug, meaning that components of living organisms are used in its production and in the final product itself. For Remicade, mouse antibody genes are utilized to compose this drug. If this confuses you, you're not alone. For years I took this medication and understood virtually nothing about what was in it, where it comes from, or how it works. Many drugs are given names you can't pronounce, and are filled with even more ingredients that you can't pronounce. I believe this is part of establishing compliance among patients.

Remicade was only approved by the FDA in 1998, and was not approved for children until 2002. There is virtually no data available on the negative long-term effects this drug could have. A great aunt of mine took Remicade for arthritis, another condition approved for treatment. She died a few years later. But because she was older anyway, there wasn't a lot of questioning among the family. I went on this medication just nine years after it was approved for children. The initial round of pediatric patients were only then approaching adulthood, but there was really no way of knowing what could have gone wrong.

For men specifically, there is reason to be concerned that conventional treatment options can negatively affect reproductive health. Research has shown that infliximab (Remicade) can decrease sperm motility, while its impacts on the quality of sperm remain unknown.[46] Worse, many men remain ignorant of this reality. Other studies have found that only one in ten men is ever counseled about these risks before beginning treatment.[47] These drugs are still recent developments and lack long-term studies or analysis on how men and their offspring may be affected.

I was never consulted on any potential harms Remicade may have on male reproductive health before starting this drug—nor were any potential dangers ever mentioned by my doctors during the decade-plus that I was on it. As I approached the age of wanting to have a family, thinking about what Remicade and all the medications I ever took did (or potentially did) started to scare the hell out of me. I was worried about what impact it might have on my future children. In addition to still being sick and wanting to take charge of my own health, I wanted to get this drug out of my body and work to mediate any harm it may have done. The themes of this book on overcoming autoimmune disease overlap with many factors that support overall male health. I must stress again that I am no doctor, but eating healthy, exercising, lifting heavy weights, and cold showers help boost testosterone—and in my judgment these and other testosterone-boosting habits can help alleviate any potential damage done to your reproductive capacity.

On its official website, Remicade boasts, "Approximately 3 out of 10 patients achieved remission with REMICADE at Week 30 compared with approximately 2 out of 10 patients not given REMICADE."[48] There is not an overwhelming difference between 30 percent and 20 percent. However, notice the word *approximately*. Was it actually 2.5 out of 10, which was then rounded up to 3? Was 2 really 2.4 and rounded down to 2? Misleading statistics, especially in the medical sphere, should not be new to most Americans. How could it? We are constantly inundated with pharma ads that present eyebrow-raising stats and figures about the efficacy of their medication. Also, thirty weeks is more than half the year, and over half the patients still were not in remission. As you'll see in a later chapter, the proper diet, exercise, spirituality, and supplement routine has a greater chance of healing you in less than half a year.

If that weren't enough, Remicade's own website lists serious infections, heart failure, liver injury, blood problems, nervous system disorders, and other potentially life-threatening side effects. For more information about specific drugs that are prescribed for Crohn's and other anti-inflammatory diseases, see the Appendix at the back of the book.

The most ironic disclaimer on many of these medications, including Remicade, is the risk of infection. As conventional medicine teaches, Crohn's disease results from your body's immune system attacking cells within the GI tract. Therefore, Remicade "works" by suppressing your body's immune system—a natural physiological function—thereby leaving you vulnerable to new infections. The job of the immune system is to fight infections. But since the immune system is the villain in Crohn's disease, it must be suppressed—at the cost of leaving you susceptible to outside infections.

In other words, the medication is not addressing the root

causes and allowing the body to heal itself without outside intervention. Functional medicine, which we will talk about later, does all of that.

Again, the purpose of clinical drugs is to achieve remission, not heal you. The natural healing approach requires more time, patience, and effort, but the results are well worth it. The satisfaction of not having any foreign substances in your body that can harm you and your offspring is incredible. The self-confidence you will gain by taking control of your health and curing your autoimmune disease is immense.

As long as you are attached to the schedule of going to doctor's appointments and taking any medicine they give you—often without question—your confidence will suffer, as you can never truly be your own person under this type of supervision from the medical experts.

WHAT THE HUMAN BODY IS CAPABLE OF

Doctors may insist that you need a certain medication, test, procedure, or even surgery to live another day. They often obsess over test results, including lab work, and are on the verge of admitting you to the ER if a single metric is one standard deviation from the norm. There are several flaws with this. For one, what does it mean to have "normal" test results in a country where being fat or obese is considered normal? What does it mean to have "normal" biomarkers when the average American consumes a diet high in ultra-processed food? What does it mean to be "normal" if the average American is taking prescription medications? What does it mean to be "normal" if the life expectancy in the US is declining and Americans are feeling lonelier, anxious, sad, and depressed?

Yet these metrics are what doctors in the US compare their

patients to. They don't account for nuance and rarely for circumstances that may cause certain biomarkers and tests to differ.

I've always been a history buff, and I am repeatedly amazed at some of the situations men of old once found themselves in. Not only did these events occur before modern medicine, but the men in many cases survived against overwhelming odds when conventional wisdom would assure you that men in such conditions must perish.

Examples exist that should raise questions about what is truly required to survive. It may not be an optimal level of vitamin D; it may rather be a testament of will and community. It may be that men who grew up in rural environments and ate real food developed such strong immune systems that their bodies were capable of handling the challenges they faced during adulthood. Equally important to point out is that their mucosal lining, brain function, testosterone levels, and overall bodily functions could not be damaged by the modern diet and the chemicals and toxins in our environment.

This has been a long-held theory of mine. It used to fascinate my family that my grandfather and his five siblings were all still living into their eighties and nineties. Not only were they living, but they were also doing well physically and mentally at a very advanced age. Although I never knew how to articulate it, it was my instinctive belief that growing up on a farm and eating the fresh fruits, vegetables, and livestock raised during their childhood throughout the 1920s and 1930s established such strong metabolic health that contributed to their longevity. They all ate junk food at times throughout their adulthood, but their intestinal fortitude was strong, and their mucosal lining was not damaged in their childhood. These were happy people and churchgoers. Mind, body, and spirit. It's how we reach old age.

By modern medical standards, the way so many people were

forced to live their lives in the early part of the country should have killed those who endured these hardships. There was no way to actually test for vitamins, minerals, white blood cells, etc. Animals cannot test for these either, but they are driven by instinct to obtain the nutrients they need by grazing or hunting for what they are lacking. A deer feeds on acorns, berries, grass, bark, flowers, and corn—all in an effort to obtain the various nutrients they instinctively know they need. We should function the same way.

In short, your body is capable of remarkable things, including healing itself. If our ancestors could survive the circumstances they dealt with in centuries past, overcoming autoimmune disease should be nothing for those of us who are affected by it. Although the majority of our food may be corrupted by manmade additives and chemicals, it has never been easier, in some ways, to eat naturally and healthily. There is an increasing number of start-up regenerative agriculture farms that offer fresh beef and eggs. When you do have to shop in a grocery store, there are more resources available to help you distinguish which foods are healthy and which ones to avoid.

It's time for Americans to question the conventional medical advice and practices they have blindly followed for years. The old way of doing things hasn't worked. Americans today are unhealthier than ever. The persistent pattern of routine appointments followed by testing and prescription hasn't served patients well. For over a decade I continued through this dead-end process, each time assured by my doctors that a change in the dose or a new blood test would fix things. My symptoms continued all the while, despite doctors insisting they had my inflammation under control. For those with Crohn's, you need to learn how to heal yourself.

You cannot count on doctors, hospitals, and prescription

drugs. It's time for something new. There are three major components to healing: faith, fitness, and nutrition. If you have an autoimmune disease and don't know where to begin, start with these.

PART TWO

HEALING YOURSELF

Chapter Four

ASK GOD TO HEAL YOU

"Bless the Lord, O my soul, and do not forget all his benefits:

Who forgives all your iniquity; who heals all your diseases."

—PSALMS 103:2–3

I believe there is a significant spiritual component to healing. If God created man in his image and gave him the earth to inhabit with all its creation, it is more than logical to begin your healing journey by asking God to heal you. It is the first step to true recovery and rediscovering your vitality. If you are willing to put in the work, He will help you become a happier, healthier version of yourself. He does not want you to be sick; He wants you to live and thrive. You are created in His image, so a sickly, weak version of you reflects poorly on Him. Yes, there are ailments that afflict people and circumstances that none of us understand. But I don't believe that a merciful God would impose a debilitating condition on anyone.

If you are in the midst of a Crohn's flare, or suffering from the symptoms of any autoimmune disease, ask God to come into your body and heal you. Welcome Him in. Surrendering your health to Him does not let you off the hook—you still have to put in the work. Rather, it makes recovering much easier. Jesus said in Matthew 7:7, "Ask, and it will be given you; search, and you will find; knock, and the door will be opened for you." Ask and pray that God will heal you. Once He is on your side in this matter, your troubles will not disappear, but you will have the most powerful ally on your side to combat them. After you help cure yourself and are living a healthy and symptom-free life, it is equally important to praise God for the good days—especially after knowing how bad it can get. This is an important point that will be developed shortly.

When working to overcome autoimmune disease naturally, you won't always have someone there to motivate you. Hopefully you do have an existing family and friend structure that can be there during these difficult times. But even then, you can't expect those closest to you to truly understand what you are going through. You cannot always rely on external factors to motivate you as you work to become drug-free. The desire to get well must come from within. This, as you know, can be the most challenging aspect of Crohn's. This point will be fleshed out in a later chapter, but for now it's important to keep in mind that He also desires you to be well.

The Bible has so much guidance on every aspect of our lives: marriage, money, and business, but also food and health. This book should be at the foundation of all your endeavors, including your health. Here it is worth repeating the three aspects of healing: nutrition, fitness, and faith. Prayer is important. But don't expect a quick fix if you are still a couch potato. Prayer is a catalyst for you to get well, but remember that you still have to put in the work. We'll kick off the triad by talking about faith and dig deeper into the spiritual component of healing.

Consider some insightful verses from scripture that can help you achieve lasting health as you battle IBD.

James 5:15 says, "The prayer of faith will save the sick, and the Lord will raise them up."

Pray to be healed. That's an important step. God does not snap His fingers and make you well all at once. You cannot eat junk food and never exercise but expect to pray and get well. Prayer alone without deliberate actions won't help. As you begin your healing journey by revamping your fitness and nutritional regimen, it's important to give God the credit as you start to see improvement.

Not only should you ask to be healed, but ask yourself why you want to be healed. Yes, no one wants to live with a life-long illness. The reasons for wanting to be symptom-free are obvious—you want to feel better! But if He grants you better health, consider how you will use that health to serve Him. At a minimum, you should live with a profound sense of gratitude once you overcome Crohn's or whatever unique health challenge you face.

After recovering from my surgery in 2019, I began the slow work of getting my body back in shape. Within six weeks, I was able to perform light body-weight exercises and use the StairMaster. Five mornings a week I was at the gym at 6:00 a.m. I gradually worked up to thirty minutes on the StairMaster on Mondays, Wednesdays, and Fridays. This was followed by a series of push-ups and pull-ups. My progress was slow, but it's amazing how fast you can build strength and endurance when you stay consistent. During my first workout back from surgery, I did three reverse-grip pull-ups, five times. I was extremely sore for days following these fifteen reps. But within a few months, I was flying through my one hundred pull-ups, two hundred push-ups morning workout. I fell in love with my new routine and was impressed by my progress. I also started doing something I had never done before in the gym: praising God.

While on the StairMaster and in between sets of pull-ups and push-ups, I found saying "thank you, God" and "thank you, Jesus" as I exercised to be immensely helpful. I meant it too. I was so grateful to be pain-free and able to exercise and move.

LET GO OF BLAME

"Heal me, O Lord, and I shall be healed; save me, and I shall be saved: for you are my praise."

—JEREMIAH 17:14

For some with autoimmune disease, the cause may be completely untraceable. Yet I believe that as you explore your own history and begin to search for the root causes, culprits will start to emerge. In Chapter 2 we described Crohn's as being triggered by external factors. This could include harmful foods you ate, chemicals, toxins, and parasites, as well as stress and trauma. I believe in stoicism as much as any real man (remember, men aren't supposed to be self-revealers!). It is not feminine, however, to acknowledge that there may be things in your past that you need to reconcile. Lingering stress, trauma, or bad memories in your head can manifest in the symptoms of IBD. When working to overcome Crohn's, it is important to forgive and move on from anything in your past.

There is a very real mental and emotional element to healing. It is crucial as you move forward in this recovery to let go of anything in your past that has prevented you from healing altogether. Learn from whatever mistakes you have made, but don't dwell on them. Only one man has ever lived a perfect life, so the rest of us have regrets of some kind. Not everything was done perfectly or planned perfectly. You had bad interactions with people. Relationships and endeavors went wrong and may have contributed to your health problems. It's okay to tuck those regrets away and learn from them, but don't let them consume your every thought and prevent you from living anew. Instead, look forward to the opportunities you have ahead of you and go forward with confidence. Listen, if you feel guilty about something in your past that is continuing to cause symptoms, forgive yourself and those involved. The only unforgivable sin is the refusal to accept Jesus as your Lord and Savior. Failing to forgive yourself and let go may be prolonging your disease.

You would wreck your car if you drove while looking at the rearview mirror the whole time. The windshield is bigger for a reason. Look forward—even if you don't always know where you are going, at least you'll see what's coming. One last point on this. If you find that your memories exceed your dreams, you are probably near the end of your life. Even if you are sick and working to overcome a diagnosis, you should still have dreams and aspirations for yourself. If you only dwell on what you believe is lost time due to years you spent sick, you'll never redirect your attention and focus to all God has for you ahead. He has so much more in store for you. Continue to have dreams and goals in the midst of your physical suffering. Once you are healed, these are yours to pursue.

RITE OF PASSAGE

Depending on how rough your experience has been, there may be times when you think that God gave you this illness to punish you. I have thought this at times, but it's not a healthy way to view your condition. Instead, learn to treat it as a challenging phase that God trusted you to handle. It should be reassuring to know that the symptoms are temporary, and a healthier version of yourself lies ahead. You may realize after dealing with Crohn's or autoimmune disease that God used this experience to teach you something about yourself. You may discover a talent or a passion, or refine your vision for life in the midst of being sick.

You will never grow as a person if you are too comfortable. That's why I believe God gives you problems to help you develop. These are challenges that you have to overcome and persevere through. Even if it takes the form of a medical diagnosis. I repeatedly make the point about my experience with Crohn's serving as a rite of passage—to become a stronger and healthier version of myself. Don't discount anything you learn about yourself during this trial; it may change your life. I would not have started exercising as soon as I did if not for Crohn's. Crohn's may have been God's wakeup call for me to finally start moving, and I feel much better since listening.

Living a Christian life requires you to step out of your comfort zone and away from what is safe. For too long, as a lukewarm believer, I took a safe, passive approach to my health. I did what was considered safe and comfortable. It wasn't until I had the courage to step out and take a leap of faith that I quit Remicade and discovered true healing. The Bible is full of examples of those who stepped away from what is comfortable—Abraham, Moses, and Ruth. If you're still struggling with autoimmune disease, it could be that you are playing life way too safe. Be bold and willing to step out and take charge of your own health.

EAT HIS FOOD

One of the primary factors that led to my diagnosis was being a junk-food addict. It may not have been God outright punishing me, but I did experience the very real consequences that sinful, gluttonous appetite can carry. The Bible teaches that gluttony is wrong. Until about six months before being diagnosed, I was very guilty of it. To be fair, part of it was ignorance. You can easily self-justify your own eating habits by thinking that anything in moderation is okay for you. However, there are some foods best avoided altogether. My diagnosis, in part, was a consequence of drifting off food-wise from the fruit and vegetables he endowed our planet with. This is an intuitive point, and more will follow in a later chapter. You instinctively know that the more candy and pizza you eat, the worse you feel. Conversely, eating a salad, an apple, or a plain potato has a substantially greater impact on your mood and health. Eat His food, not our food.

The explosion in autoimmune diseases has coincided with the period when Americans have moved away from God and the Church. But they have not moved away in just a religious sense; Americans have also become more disconnected from the land itself, and the food it produces.

The acupuncturist I saw early into my diagnosis told me the human body has the potential to live to be 130 years old. It sounds unbelievable at first. But then consider examples from the Bible. The Old Testament is filled with men and women who achieved incredible longevity. For example, Jacob lived to be 117. Joseph lived to be 110. Abraham and Sarah lived to be 175 and 127, respectively. How did they do it? Faith in their Creator for sure, but they also had the benefit of consuming the food God endowed the earth with in its raw, unpolluted, and uncorrupted state. What foods do they mention in the Bible? Not Pizza Rolls and potato chips. Those in Bible times consumed lamb, fish, beef, wheat, figs, olives, and honey. To be sure, natural diets vary slightly based on geography, but they consumed what God put on this earth, and even then, not everything was fair game. There were Biblical restrictions placed on what people could eat back then, such as shellfish and swine.

When the Lord spoke to Moses and Aaron in Leviticus Chapter 11, he instructed them on what to eat, saying:

From among all the land animals, these are the creatures that you may eat.

Any animal that has divided hoofs and is cleft-footed and chews the cud—such you may eat.

God gives us the green light to eat beef! God then rules out creatures such as the camel, rock badger, and pig as animals that his people should not eat. Nuance plays a significant role in the treatment of Crohn's and autoimmune diseases, and this is especially important when considering diet, which will be addressed in a later chapter. Not every food or food restriction is for everyone. The big takeaway is to have boundaries and dietary limits. Treat your body like a temple and be very selective about what you allow inside. You may find that following Leviticus Chapter 11 to the letter will help you in your healing journey, and spiritual journey as well.

To be sure, there are also several contemporary examples of people who reach old age, not just living to their late nineties but to one hundred and beyond. More often than not, centenarians have three dominant characteristics in their lives: strong family ties, an agrarian background, and faithful church attendance. Again, mind, body, and spirit are the keys to longevity and greater health.

When it comes to what you eat, it is also important to consider how to eat.

Moreover, it is God's gift that all should eat and drink and take pleasure in all their toil.

—ECCLESIASTES 3:13

For even when we were with you, we gave you this command: Anyone unwilling to work should not eat.

—2 THESSALONIANS 3:10

There is something especially unhealthy about the American way of eating. For most of human history, eating was a reward for your work. It required a great physical effort just to prepare something to eat. Raising the cow, milking the cow, butchering the cow, cooking the beef, plowing the field, sowing the wheat, reaping the wheat, milling the wheat into flour. You can quickly grasp how difficult the process of eating was, and still is, for a lot of people around the world. With the exception of modern-day homesteaders, and religious or ethnic communities who have made or are making a conscious effort to return to this lifestyle, many Americans enjoy food as a convenience. Food is readily available in the refrigerator, pantry, local grocery store, or fast-food restaurant. Food has become a social habit for many. There is something very unfulfilling, however, about eating for its own sake; about consuming ultra-processed food just for the sake of wanting to eat something—without having done anything to deserve it.

I used to be, in effect, the yard boy for my grandparents. Maintaining the grass, weeds, tree limbs, sticks, and more on a large yard in the country could easily fill up your Saturday. My grandmother used to cook a delicious meal for my grandfather and me upon my completion. Usually baked chicken, green beans, and rice. Eating good home-cooked food never tastes better than it does after hours of physical work outside. Eating after working on a computer all day isn't nearly as fulfilling. It's one of the reasons I love to wake up early and have a great morning workout. Eating in the morning tastes so much better if you start your day with an hour of exercise.

The point is that the Bible teaches us that food is meant to fuel our bodies. Food is consumed as a reward for work, and should not be eaten for its own sake. Most of us are still guilty of eating for fun, and there are times to just enjoy. But let this be the exception, not the rule.

There is a tremendous satisfaction I experience when eating really healthy, or not eating at all and enjoying a fast. Your body has the chance to reset, detoxify, and remain fallow. Your head becomes clearer. If you ever dare to venture back into the ultra-processed food market, you will notice the difference immediately when placing that food in your mouth. The temples in your head become warm, your mouth feels gross, and your brain becomes muddy. Imagine then, the calming effect that healthy eating can have for you.

And the Lord God commanded the man, saying, You may freely eat of every tree of the garden.

—GENESIS 2:16

We don't know precisely what the forbidden fruit was. But we do have God's instruction that "of every tree" you may eat its fruit, other than the Tree of Life, of course. With the exception of the Forbidden Fruit, virtually any seed-bearing plant is fair game. These are the foods God intended for us. Many Biblical scholars now believe that there was no such thing as a carnivore until the Fall of Man. This includes animals. There were no meat-eating lions and dinosaurs until man sinned. I do not believe there is an explicit call for mankind to return to the vegetarian diet, but there is a lesson to be learned. For those with active IBD, one of the first things you will do is immediately change your diet. Meat is usually a good food to drop in the midst of a flare; instead, opt for beef broth, chicken broth, or bone broth. This allows the gut to heal and regain the ability to handle foods like beef and poultry again. Fruits and vegetables, cooked to ensure manageable digestion, are a go-to in times of active symptoms.

If my people who are called by my name humble themselves, pray, seek my face, and turn from their wicked ways, then I will hear from heaven and will forgive their sin and heal their land.

—2 CHRONICLES 7:14

At the risk of taking this verse out of context, God gives us an interesting phrase to ponder in "heal their land." Now, He is referring to the people of Israel and asking them to look to him and abandon the idols of the earth. One reason for the explosion in autoimmune diseases has been the increased use of pesticides, fertilizers, and other chemicals used in growing our food. Unfortunately, these man-made additives remain in the ground—corrupting future growth whether or not new fertilizers are applied. As a part of the effort to make Americans healthy, emphasis has been put on the often-overlooked component of restoring the soil. This will require time, money, and commitment from landowners and policymakers, but it's a necessary endeavor to improve overall health.

HEAL IN FELLOWSHIP

Healing yourself can sometimes be a long and lonely process. You cannot expect anyone to understand, or even truly care about, what you are going through. This can be an especially difficult reality for IBD patients. A strong community of support is vital to overcoming any challenge. Yet the insecurity caused by IBD can create self-induced isolation for fear of symptoms attacking while in a social setting. I struggled with this for years, making the liberating feeling of finally becoming drug-free all the more profound. If you feel that no one will listen to you regarding your symptoms, let me assure you that He is there for you to help you overcome your autoimmune disease. You can always talk to God during these times. There is no voicemail with Him. Open up to Him about your health problems and seek His help. From the Word, here are some passages that directly call on the need for others:

Are any among you sick? They should call for the elders of the church and have them pray over them, anointing them with oil in the name of the Lord.

—JAMES 5:14

Therefore confess your sins to one another and pray for one another, so that you may be healed. The prayer of the righteous is powerful and effective.

—JAMES 5:16

Having a strong social group is vital for your health. We're social creatures and need other people. With Crohn's, I was often too embarrassed to go out and socialize. My symptoms continued and persisted as long as I was lonely. This was a painful paradox to confront. Having been sick during my coming-of-age years, and failing to establish strong, meaningful friendships, I continued to lack the socialization that I desperately wanted. And consequently, I was still sick. With no one to talk to at Troy, I dove deeper into the Word. I did a bunch of journaling while I worked to heal myself and had many one-on-one conversations with God. It felt good, and I started to see the results. As my symptoms improved, I got more comfortable in my own skin. This made socialization more possible for a change. While the Bible gives rare examples of loneliness being necessary before important events, it's not intended for most of us, and not a natural condition to find ourselves in. Yet if you do find yourself isolated, try to use this situation to your advantage. I didn't ask for a season of loneliness, but God gave me one for the purpose of overcoming Crohn's—to focus on healing myself and to salvage the rest of my existence.

Having a community is vital to your overall well-being, and church is a great place to start. In 2020, many churches were shut down or operated remotely. This contributed to the social isolation many experienced and the subsequent wave of health problems that developed or went undetected. This likely exacerbated the socialization problems that can trouble IBD patients. As I began my natural recovery from Crohn's, I instantly realized that I had let this disease hold me back in so many ways over the years, especially personally and socially.

One of the most impactful things you can do for your health is to reestablish, or build from scratch, a strong social group. Early into my diagnosis, there were often hospital advertisements for support groups. This never appealed to me. I didn't want to dwell in agony with others over our collective troubles. I just wanted to be able to do normal activities with a great group of people. The gym and Bible study groups became my most prolific social outlets.

Despite the few examples of isolation, the Bible also teaches and makes a stronger case for the importance of a strong community and fellowship. It's how we grow and handle the challenges that come our way. Among the first actions Jesus took was to establish a group of friends, his disciples, to help with his ministry. Indeed, the church itself is a community of believers. If you have neglected this aspect of your well-being because of an autoimmune disease, I urge you to prioritize building relationships with people. It can be difficult at first, especially if the insecurity from IBD lingers, but once you start, your confidence will steadily improve. I was amazed when so many of my symptoms vanished when I finally had a good group of people to consistently surround myself with. We are not meant to be lone rangers. We need companionship and a strong social circle.

God didn't create Adam to be sick, but to tend the Garden of Eden. Adam was to care for the animals and cultivate the garden and its abundant produce. He was not put on earth to spend his days taking medicine or plagued with chronic illness. After all, how could he work if that were the case? The desire to become drug-free is inherently spiritual. It is not bashing the doctors and healthcare workers. But it is trusting your own instinctive feeling that God does not want a permanently sick version of you. Don't put your faith in Big Pharma, put it in God.

Mankind was created in the image of God. That includes you. Therefore, everything you do with your body, put in your body, and say with your body must be done in a manner that honors and pleases Him. Yes, we all fall short and have our own struggles. But the goal is to strive to always live a life that glorifies God. The food you eat, the decision to exercise, and the thoughts you have all determine your state of health. When it comes to becoming healthier and overcoming your incurable autoimmune disease, understand this: A sickly, weak version of yourself does not reflect well on Him or you. Once you have decided to get healthy and transform your body, thank God and praise Him for the desire to be healthy, for the desire and ability to move and become the fittest, most active version of yourself.

Chapter Five

MOVE LIKE A PRIMITIVE MAN

"If you obey nature's laws, you can be born again."

—PAUL BRAGG

Art from antiquity can reveal many things about our present society. One of my favorite pieces is the statue *Laocoön and His Sons*, which depicts an outstretched Laocoön grappling with a sea serpent. His muscles are strained, the bicep vein in his left arm popping out like a rope, while his abdomen, chest, and quads show impressive definition—the way you would expect an ancient Greek to look. Art in any healthy society will depict the most beautiful things, both people and nature. Yet even when accounting for any exaggeration the sculptor may have added, the contrast is stark compared to contemporary times.

American men are failing in many respects. There are economic challenges, deaths of despair, and men lagging behind women educationally. These occurrences are unfortunate and should not be dismissed as minor hiccups in the well-being of males overall in America. Among the most profound changes in American men, indeed the most visible and obvious, is how the physical condition has deteriorated in recent decades. The now-common sightings of fat men are disturbing when you consider what it means to the health of the nation overall. It is a sign of a bad diet, poor food quality, a lack of personal pride in maintaining one's appearance—which can indicate a life void of purpose and meaning to allow oneself to deteriorate into such a physical state.

Your weight and physical shape significantly determine your overall well-being, especially your mental state. This is not to explicitly fat-shame men and women. On the contrary, I commend and encourage our heavy friends in the gym who are making a sincere effort to live healthier lives. But the problem seems almost out of hand. The "dad bod" has been completely normalized, leading many young men to neglect their physical shape and allow a coat of fat to form on their midsection. As one of my more candid uncles describes the phenomenon, "These men are building a shed over their tool." Drinking beer, eating chips, and devouring fried foods—usually while seated and watching a ball game—have become normalized to the point where they are the new seminal American male activity.

This trend needs to be reversed for society as a whole and especially for those with autoimmune diseases. Being overweight is a leading indicator of so many health problems. The solution to curing or preventing a host of health problems lies in addressing your weight. In the aftermath of my initial diagnosis, I found exercise to be a godsend. Exercise provided so many benefits, including a boost to my self-esteem and gradual improvements to my physique. But more fundamentally, it just felt good to move.

THE KEYSTONE TO HEALTH

In America, and throughout the West, medicine has shifted from preventative care designed to keep you healthy (a proactive approach) to a reactive, sick-care approach that emphasizes treating patients who are already sick. It's time for a health revolution to restore the old medical practice of preventative care, of which fitness is a crucial element.

For thousands of years, exercise has been known to be the keystone to a person's health. The emphasis on health rather than disease goes back to the classics and was taught by physicians of the ancient world, including Hippocrates and Galen. Hippocrates allegedly said, "Eating alone will not keep a man well; he must also take exercise."[49]

Galen structured his medical theory around the naturals and non-naturals. "Central to this theory was health and the uses and abuses of the 'six things nonnatural:' 1) air, 2) food and drink (diet), 3) sleep and waking, 4) motion (exercise) and rest, 5) excretions and retentions, and 6) passions of the mind. If the non-naturals were observed and practiced in moderation, health would be the result. But if not followed, performed in excess, or put into imbalance, disease or illness would result."[50] In so many ways, the modern functional medicine approach is simply a rediscovery of what the ancients, including Galen, already knew.

Motion and rest, as taught by ancient physicians, meant exercise, and this remained fundamental to personal well-being in the medical literature through the late 1800s. Furthermore, the ancients taught that everyone had agency over their own health—it was not preordained by the Gods who would be healthy and who would be sick. "Every person, either independently or in counsel with their physician, had the opportunity to attain and preserve health."[51] This is an especially important concept to keep in mind if you have Crohn's and autoimmune disease. Yes, we may have gotten our diagnosis because we carried a genetic propensity to get it. Despite this genetic propensity and the environmental factors that contributed to it, the ability to heal yourself is still within reach.

By the 18th century, ancient principles on hygiene and regimen continued to be upheld in Europe, especially in regard to exercise. For instance, in Scottish physician William Buchan's highly popular *Domestic Medicine*, first published in 1769, he suggested that "of all the causes which conspire to render the lives of children short and miserable, none has greater influence than the want of proper exercise."[52]

A conscious effort to become healthy in America began in the late nineteenth century, as growing cities and populations produced poor sanitation and living conditions that resulted in adverse health outcomes. Moreover, the lack of space to move outdoors gave rise to the concept of gymnasiums, the YMCA, and New York's Downtown Athletic Club, for instance. As the country became more settled and civilized, there gave rise to collegiate sports. Unlike men in other nations frequently engaged in war, young men in America were free to use their masculine energy on the gridiron and ballfield. Sports permeated the playground and schoolyard, and soon every boy in America knew how to throw a baseball.

While sports are not inherently bad, the emphasis on sports misses the whole point. Athletes were conditioned to be in shape, but the rest of the student body at schools and universities was neglected. I used to believe that all American men were stout and strong up until the 1950s and 1960s. I was shocked to learn, however, that one-third of the men drafted for World War I were deemed physically unfit for service.[53] If men were beginning to decline physically in the early 1900s, the problem has only grown exponentially since.

Fitness icon Jack LaLanne further popularized the modern health movement. LaLanne even invented several pieces of now-common gym equipment. Moreover, American public schools began implementing rigorous exercise programs to help keep America's youth healthy and fit. It would seem as if the country was laying the groundwork for a future filled with health nuts. Today, fitness centers are popular destinations, and it's refreshing to see them so well used.

The YMCA, Gold's Gym, and Planet Fitness have become household names across the country. Yet despite the prevalence of gyms and a greater understanding of science, Americans at large remain an inactive and unhealthy bunch.

The benefits of exercise to those with IBD are self-evident. For example, new academic literature highlights the benefits of strength training for Crohn's patients, as this disease can lead to bone loss. One recent study highlighted the problem of bone loss in Crohn's patients. There are several reasons for this, including nutritional deficiency and problems with nutrient absorption.

According to the paper, "There have been a number of studies examining the prevalence of osteopenia and osteoporosis in Crohn's disease with reports that up to 80% of CD patients suffer from some degree of bone loss."[54] Osteoporosis is defined as "a loss of bone mass and the micro-architectural deterioration of bone tissue leading to a subsequent increase in bone fracture." Crohn's patients may be especially susceptible as several factors associated with the disease, such as chronic inflammation, inadequate nutrition, and genetic susceptibility to bone loss, can all contribute to the development of osteoporosis.[55]

The role of exercise in treating Crohn's has received little attention from conventional providers. But it's not ignored in this paper, as the authors find that "high impact exercise and activities that produce large muscle forces may have a positive impact on skeletal health in patients with CD."[56]

Based on my experience, I found exercise to be one of the quickest ways to recover from a flare and hospitalization. When you start exercising, it almost seems like your body understands that it's not allowed to be sick anymore. Your body locks in and knows that it's time to start doing healthy things once again. If you've been sick and in the hospital, your body may tell you something like this: *We just experienced a setback, but now I'm ready to start moving again.* These are some of the insights I've learned from using fitness to overcome Crohn's.

WIN THE MORNING

Few things are less manly than grown men complaining about having to wake up early. Men are not supposed to be idle and lazy. They are to wake early and attack the day. "Win the morning" has been another long-held maxim of mine. I believe you should wake up early, ideally without an alarm clock, put your feet on the floor, and start moving. An alarm clock may be set as a precaution, but once your body clock is in tune with your new schedule, you should find yourself beating the alarm most mornings.

I wake up at 4:30 a.m. on weekdays to begin my exercise routine. I change up my morning workouts every few months to keep it new. I'll go through phases where I stick to cardio and core in the mornings, and train with weights in the afternoon. I have always loved doing bodyweight exercises in the morning and usually incorporate some variation of these. Some people love to wake up early and enjoy quiet Bible time first thing. I have tried this at times, but always find it hard to sit still after waking up. I'm ready to move and will exercise for at least an hour every morning.

This chapter is about exercise, but I wouldn't be giving you all the information if I didn't talk about sleep. Great workouts start with great sleep. Unfortunately, many Americans struggle through the night. If you haven't experienced it yourself, you have surely met people who claim they "can't sleep." It is my contention that many struggle to fall asleep because they lack the discipline to put their phones down—the algorithms in apps and on the web aggressively work to keep them hooked—and are constantly stimulated by the light reflected from these or other screens. Have the discipline to put the screens away an hour or two before going to bed. Secondly, they have not done enough hard things throughout the day. They hit the pillow and can instantly tell that they did not exhaust all or even half the energy in their body. In other words, sometimes not being able to fall asleep could be an indictment of yourself—that you did not exercise or work hard throughout your waking hours. If your day was too easy, if you are too comfortable, a lack of sleep may be the consequence.

One often takes care of the other. If you struggle to sleep and don't exercise, you may find that starting an exercise routine will instantly help you with your sleep. Additionally, it's really important for your body to adopt a strong sleep pattern. Strive to be in bed at the same time each night and wake up roughly at the same time each morning. Even on weekends, my sleep schedule is rarely off by more than thirty minutes, either going to bed or waking up. As with the rest of this book, the importance of sleep is intuitive.

Sleep is when your body is allowed to rest and repair, to build muscle and grow. For those with Crohn's and autoimmune disease, it's when real healing happens. Although there are numerous studies and medical experts hailing its importance, you know how crucial sleep is to your wellbeing. Early into my diagnosis, I found sleeping very difficult. There is stomach pain that keeps you up, and repeated trips to the bathroom during the night. Thankfully, these sleep problems didn't persist, only while my Crohn's was active. When I was still with Vanderbilt, I participated in a study examining how well Crohn's patients slept. I was able to sleep fine by this point, and I don't recall any issues. Sleep is a good indicator of how well you are handling Crohn's or colitis. While experiencing symptoms, it is difficult to make it through the night—either due to pain or bathroom trips, or both. So, if you are able to sleep through the night, pain-free, and without having to go to the bathroom, this is a great indicator of your overall health and your ability to overcome these symptoms.

I have to leave room for nuance. It's important to listen to your body. If you need more sleep, then sleep. If your body is recovering from a flare and hospitalization, sleep. I have also noticed, though, that sometimes forcing your body to get back into rhythm is the quickest way to recovery.

I am thrilled to wake up at 4:30 in the morning with no pain and ready to attack the day. The sense of accomplishment after a great workout completed as the sun is just starting to shine is unreal. Importantly, you cannot control everything that happens during the day. But you can control what time you get up and what you do during your first few hours. Get up and win the morning.

EXERCISE AND RECOVERY

Without exercise, it is doubtful that I ever would have recovered from my initial near-fatal spell with Crohn's in 2009. In the worst possible physical shape of my life, I became determined to build a better body. I was tired of being weak, tired of having a pudgy stomach and scrawny arms. This may sound silly given my physical shape, but my goal was to achieve six-pack abs. I had never lifted a weight or even been good at gym class in elementary school, but I wanted to turn this most troublesome portion of my body into something I could be proud of.

I resolved to get healthy, get in shape, and build some muscle. I had virtually no guidance on how to begin a fitness regimen, so I did what seemed logical: I got outside and started walking. As winter turned to spring, then summer, I found so much solace and enjoyment in walking. Walking soon gave way to running, and many miles were traveled every day on foot after school. Walking and running led to an interest in building strength, and I began doing push-ups and ab exercises. Even more inspiration was found when I learned about Herschel Walker and how he transformed his body from a plump child into a muscular All-American tailback without the use of weights. If push-ups and sit-ups could do it for Herschel, they could do it for me too. I was getting stronger, and my fragile body began to change. I didn't become the next Herschel Walker, but I wasn't the sick kid in the hospital bed either.

To truly take my newfound love for fitness to the next level, I had to start lifting weights. At the time, lifting weights still seemed like an unattainable reality given my age, shape, and resources. Fortunately, the opportunity to play high school football introduced me to the vaunted weight room, and I was lucky to learn the basics from some much stronger older players. The gym has become a constant in my life and has been extremely beneficial for overcoming Crohn's.

My fitness routine started in isolation, just walking, running, and doing calisthenics at home. Some may prefer a home workout, but I find training at a gym to be the best way to exercise. Obviously, a gym will have more and better equipment that wouldn't be practical for most people to keep at home. There is always the question of motivation for those starting to live a healthier life. In overcoming autoimmune disease, the motivation comes from the desire to get healthier, to feel better, and to express your gratitude for doing so. Most of us still have days when we struggle to find that spark. When you exercise at a gym, you can feed off the energy of others and get inspired to push yourself further than you ever would alone. One of the main benefits of exercising in a gym or wellness center is the people you can meet. It offers the opportunity to glean insights from those more advanced than you. Several men in the gym have provided a lot of good advice and encouragement over the years—whether it was to help with a specific movement, tips for training a certain muscle, or just a kind word of inspiration.

GETTING THE MOST OUT OF EXERCISE

The pain and trauma caused by Crohn's disease and surgery can unknowingly promote wellness. All men need a rite of passage—a form of suffering in order to grow physically, mentally, and spiritually. A Crohn's flare can certainly do that. Once you are pain-free, there will be a tremendous urge to finally move, as you are free from the confines of a hospital bed and gown.

After experiencing the overwhelming pain Crohn's can unleash on the body, I am so thankful to wake up every day feeling great. When I started out, I never needed music or headphones to work out. I never needed to listen to audiobooks, motivational speeches, or podcasts in order to go hard in the gym. I was driven by a desire to be as fit and healthy as I could, never wanting to return to that helpless feeling of being unable to stand or crouch down in agony.

As you strive to become drug-free in treating IBD or your

other chronic health problems, take up exercise as an active part of this process. Exercise has many positive benefits for someone with an autoimmune disease, and taking the right approach makes a big difference.

BUILDING CONFIDENCE

The symptoms caused by autoimmune disease may have caused you at times to think negatively of yourself. They have for me. I know the feeling of being weak and helpless while hospitalized and sick. I know the feeling of being almost disgusted with my own appearance—as either a shriveled collection of skin and bones or having a scarred stomach after the surgeon's handiwork. This poor self-image can wreck your confidence, which in itself has detrimental consequences for your health.

Self-improvement through working out and training hard in the gym is one of the best ways to improve your physical condition and rebuild your confidence. It is especially beneficial when you pick specific fitness goals, work toward them, and finally achieve them. Accomplishing goals builds confidence. Lifting weights builds confidence. Pay attention as you progress in the gym and start to notice a difference in your appearance. Being unsure of your abilities is characteristic of lacking confidence. Exercise offers the best remedy, as there are multiple ways to improve your abilities. If you can't do a pull-up, train and get that first one. Ten pounds may have seemed too heavy when you just started out. In a few weeks' time, ten pounds will be lighter than your warm-up weight. As these accomplishments add up, you'll start to feel more confident in yourself and your newfound abilities. For someone who is physically weak or recovering from an illness, any workout or exercise may seem impossible. But as you start in the gym, these previously intimidating machines and weights become easier, and you'll seek new challenges. Crohn's can be such a frustrating obstacle. Setting physical challenges as goals, and then hitting them, does wonders for your confidence and recovery.

CHALLENGE YOURSELF

Remember this: What doesn't challenge you won't change you. Muscle growth occurs when you hit failure—meaning you have exhausted yourself on a set of repetitions for a particular exercise. It comes when you are making wild faces and gritting your teeth to complete the final reps. I won't get into the full anatomy and science of muscle growth. To simplify, after breaking down your muscles on these final reps, they repair and grow back even stronger. Your workouts need to be rigorous enough to push yourself, but you also cannot make yourself miserable. This will lead to burnout and the end of your fitness journey. Few things are more annoying in the gym than hearing "gym bros" complain about the next exercise or workout they have to perform. There are hundreds of movements and variations to train most muscle groups.

If you don't like one, try another. For instance, if barbell squats give you back trouble, try leg press or dumbbell squats. The immense gratitude and appreciation you will have for living a pain-free life cannot be replicated, and you'll find little to complain about in the gym or elsewhere in life once you are symptom-free.

The benefits of exercise for those with Crohn's, UC, or IBS are profound. An incredible amount of healing can be achieved through movement, especially in the aftermath of being sick, which is often associated with a lack of exercise. Many doctors will want you to rest and recover for as long as possible. Then, when they deem you fit to return to regular exercise, it can be done only for short intervals, and every iteration must be done gradually. "Don't overdo it" is the medical examiner's instruction for exercise. Now, if you have just had surgery, by all means take the appropriate time to recover. Depending on the severity of the procedure, this could take a few weeks to several months or even a year. For me, I was very determined to get active as soon as I could and started walking as much as possible within three days. Within six weeks I was doing pull-ups.

Your doctors may urge caution, and some of it is well-founded. But if your body has been through the fire of a Crohn's flare or bad UC spell, and you suddenly feel the urge to exercise, I say go for it. Ignore the professional teachings of gradualism. The faster you get back into movement, the faster you will heal. Again, your body is meant to move.

CREATE YOUR ROUTINE

When it comes to fitness, find your niche. Find the exercises you love to do and do them. Choose the movements that you truly enjoy to train each muscle. If you love walking, walk. Cycling? Cycle. Swimming? Swim. Weights? Lift. HIIT? Do it. A certain exercise or method of training may give you the fitness bug. But once you are hooked, your training will likely evolve over time to include movements, routines, or classes you never considered.

It is also important to have a balanced routine, meaning train every muscle group. Don't be the stereotypical gym rat who only trains his upper body and skips legs (or vice versa, if that's ever been done). All of your muscles need exercise. I train each muscle group twice a week and find that forty-eight hours is usually sufficient for recovery. Depending on the intensity of your routine, more or less rest may be required. For instance, if you train your chest and deplete your pectoral muscles, you might wait seventy-two hours or more before training your chest again. You can train abs like any other muscle group, once or twice a week. Once you build up your core strength, you can train your core every day.

How much should you exercise? That depends on you. To start, I am not an exercise minimalist. I believe in intentional movement every single day. This could be weight training, calisthenics, or cardio. I walk at least once a day, especially when the weather is beautiful. Walking is how I got my start, and I believe in walking in almost all kinds of weather—even when it is sweltering hot or freezing cold. I'm not suggesting that you should push yourself for hours in these extreme conditions, but try fifteen or twenty minutes in the ultra-hot sun. In the wintertime, bundle up and see if you can make it fifteen or twenty minutes in the cold. Once your body is acclimated to the weather and the habit of needing to go on a walk, these "extreme" outdoor conditions will seem less severe, and you'll look forward to the change-up in temperature. Moving in the extreme heat or cold adds an extra therapeutic layer to the walk, as your body feels especially rejuvenated after the physical challenge.

Finally, write down your routine and stick to it. Take note of your progress and fitness accomplishments. Understand, too, that results take time. The only shortcut is to stay consistent and committed.

WEIGHT LIFTING

The benefits of lifting heavy weights are known to include increased testosterone and muscle mass. Although I never had this tested while with Vanderbilt, it seems intuitive that men with autoimmune disease may naturally have less testosterone. There are many reasons for this. If you have IBD, your body may not be able to tolerate or absorb nutrients from red meat and other foods necessary for maintaining healthy testosterone levels. As you work to become drug-free, it is crucial to establish high, healthy levels of testosterone. Lifting heavy and doing hard exercises can help.

Steve Reeves and other bodybuilders or professional athletes may have certain lifting principles to help them minimize their time in the gym. This may be necessary for you depending on your work schedule and needs. It is important to rest muscle groups after training them; you have to give them a chance to recover and grow. Your training split can be divided as necessary to minimize the number of days you take completely off.

A weightlifting split can be as simple as training the upper body one day and the lower body the next, followed by a rest day. Then repeat the split to give you four days of weightlifting, Monday through Friday, with a day of rest in the middle. Others prefer to divide their weightlifting schedule into push and pull days, which entails dividing their training based on whether the movement requires a push or a pull. For example, pull-ups and pull-downs on a cable machine are pull movements. So, too, are hamstring curls and bicep curls. Push movements include triceps extensions, bench press, and shoulder press.

Still, other training splits are as straightforward as dividing the body into its major muscle groups and allocating one day a week to each. There are countless experts who swear by their routine and methods. You can find books and YouTube videos galore promoting different splits and training methods. If you are just starting out, my best advice is to just start. Just get in the gym and start lifting weights. You can figure out your perfect routine once you become acclimated to the various weights and machines your gym offers. It may take a few years, but don't wait for the perfect plan before you begin. Hiring a personal trainer can also be a great asset as you start your weight training journey. They can work with you to customize your routine based on your goals and starting point.

While some may insist on a true, literal rest day, I believe in moving every day. This is not to say that you should max out on bench press five days in a row—of course your performance on this lift would suffer if you did something like that. I always take at least one day off, sometimes two, from lifting weights each week. Even on days when I don't lift—I call these active recovery days—I'll go for a long walk, a jog, or swim. There is always some exercise to do, even if it is not in the gym.

CARDIOVASCULAR TRAINING

Some in the gym will skip cardio or advise against it, not wanting to shed weight and endanger the muscle mass they have acquired. Cardiovascular exercise consists of movement that trains your most important muscle, the heart. Your cardiovascular system includes your heart, veins, and arteries. It's the network that pumps blood throughout your body, providing oxygen to cells and removing waste. With the rise of cardiovascular disease and other heart-related health problems, it's not just IBD patients who need to train this muscle. It's as simple as moving your body, whether you go for a brisk walk or a rigorous session on the StairMaster. I found my start in fitness through cardio and would never advise skimping on this critical component. Think about humans in early times. Men were required to walk, march, or run for miles as part of their daily life. Whether in search of food or to wage war, Roman legions and other armies throughout history may have had to march twenty or more miles a day, requiring cardio stamina. The following day, these same soldiers may have had to construct a series of fortifications or fight a battle hand-to-hand, requiring the strength of their arms.

Just training for strength is a new idea that a lot of men want to follow, but you must have both the endurance to perform cardio and the strength to lift weights. The goal of fitness is to use it, not just train and train and train. Find practical applications—specifically outdoors—to test your strength and progress. For example, in the summertime I get outside, barefoot and shirtless. Find a tree to do pull-ups on and run or walk in between sets. Going on a hike, swimming, or building something outdoors are all great applications. Not only are these testing your strength, but they are all challenges with the satisfaction of accomplishment in the end.

EXERCISE TRAPS

If you are recovering from autoimmune disease and new to fitness, beware that the internet is now filled with thousands and thousands of fitness experts and influencers—all of whom swear by their own unique methodology. Many people make the dreadful mistake of comparing themselves to the models and influencers they see online, failing to realize that they are looking at edited images, heavy users, and paid professionals. You can be especially susceptible to this awful trap if you are a beginner. Don't waste time comparing yourself to others.

In your fitness journey, remember that you are competing against yourself. Compare your progress to yourself, not to others. Are you getting stronger? Do you see changes in the mirror or on the scale? Are you doing better today than you were this time last year? Are you lifting heavier weights than you were a few months ago? Are you walking or running a bit faster and farther than you were the last time you really pushed yourself? That's how you should measure yourself. Track your progress and note the steady improvement over time.

Another common exercise trap you should avoid is the euphemism of training to maintain. There is no such thing as maintaining. Every day you are either getting stronger or weaker. If you are doing the same thing you did last month, you are a weaker version of yourself today. There will be setbacks. Injuries happen. Symptoms reappear. Soreness may limit your next workout. A downpour will cancel your plans to run or walk outside. The key is how you respond to these setbacks. The goal is to come back stronger.

If you become complacent and train to maintain your present physical shape, you'll stop growing—physically, mentally, and as a person in general. Don't misunderstand me—I believe there is a big difference between being complacent and being content, perhaps one of the biggest distinctions society has misconstrued. Contentment is a positive state of mind in regard to certain aspects of life. It signals that you are comfortable in your own skin, are not jealous or envious of others, and appreciate all you have earned or been given. It means being grateful for the little things and pleased with your position in this world. Fitness-wise, it means to be grateful for the equipment you have to exercise with, whether it's a state-of-the-art weight room or the floor in your room to do push-ups on. To be complacent, by contrast, means settling for the bare minimum—when doing three pull-ups has become easy and you refuse to do a fourth.

I acknowledge that incrementalism has its limits. No one could add five pounds to a curl bar each week, year after year—there would be guys curling thousands of pounds if that were the case. The human body has limits. Pushing yourself doesn't always mean lifting the heaviest weight in the gym. It does mean exerting yourself, getting extra reps when you think you're done, or maintaining proper form as the sets get increasingly difficult. Continue to monitor your progress only against the old version of you, not others.

There will be periods, maybe a few days or a whole month, when you find yourself in a fitness funk. You'll lack the energy to lift weights or the motivation to continue. You may notice a poor mindset setting in and frustration about losing your mojo in the gym. These episodes happen, and more often than not, they are relapses of your Crohn's or autoimmune symptoms. If you notice that your routine and efforts in the gym seem out-of-whack, it's important to take inventory of your recent eating habits, sleep habits, and thoughts. It could be time to change up your routine or enjoy some nature therapy—take a break from the gym for a few days or a week while you spend your time outside in the woods, mountains, or at the beach.

My theory is twofold. Sometimes your body tells you it truly needs a break; in that case, listen. Or, if you usually exercise by yourself, your mindset can start to break down—find a partner to train with. This usually adds instant relief to your fitness routine and newfound inspiration to push yourself harder and further. Keep in mind, too, that your mental well-being plays a significant role in IBD and Crohn's. If your mindset is weak and keeps you from exercising at your usual standards, focus on fixing it immediately. It could be that you've let yourself slide nutritionally, or there is unresolved stress building up inside you. Resolve this for your own good. Keep yourself well so you can continue to exercise; it's a vital component of remaining drug-free.

THE SUM OF YOUR CHOICES

What you look like today was decided largely by what you chose to eat over the last ten years. It was decided by whether you exercised or not over the same time period. The flip side is this: What you look like in ten years—or whether you are even alive in ten years—will be determined by your dietary and fitness choices over the coming decade. If you haven't been living a healthy lifestyle, start now. If you feel you are now too old to receive any benefit from changing your diet and routine, you're not. As long as you are alive, you can choose to live a healthy life.

If you are unhappy with your current results, transform that dissatisfaction into energy to change what you see. Create a vision for what you want your body to look and feel like, and then work to make it happen. That was crucial for me while overcoming Crohn's. It was time to create a version of myself I could be proud of and erase the sick and weak version of myself. I'll talk about this in a later chapter, but your mindset is the key to tremendous healing power. If you believe you are going to be sick, you are going to be sick. If you believe you will be healthy, you will be healthy.

I have often wondered how many people who are diagnosed with cancer, or another serious health condition, received their diagnosis days or years after telling themselves "I'm probably going to get cancer." Then, with the mindset of a medical defeatist, their body took that into account and planned on getting cancer one day. Approach the gym and your workout with a positive mindset. Your results and health will notice.

TRAINING WITH WHAT YOU HAVE

My training philosophy was always simple: Do what you can with what you have. In the early days, I had the floor in my room, the grass outside, and roads in my neighborhood. I began an intense series of calisthenics to train my abs. I wanted to turn the section of my body that had given me so much trouble into something strong. Gradually, principles of strength training and exercise justified the idea of core strength. As I came to learn, core strength is critical not only for overall health, but also because it is a prerequisite for virtually every other exercise, sport, or fitness endeavor you can pursue.

Genetics and circumstances should never be used as an excuse for why you can't get to where you want to go. Yes, it may be frustrating to see some guys explode in the gym with seemingly minimal effort, or guys who have the means to employ a trainer and have the nutritional component down with serious and top-notch meal preparation. But understand where you started from. You may have just been released from the hospital and be in the worst physical shape of your life. In this condition, your goal is to rebuild yourself, not to look like someone else. As you gradually recover, your goal should be to become a stronger version of yourself. Be proud of your efforts in the gym, and don't get discouraged if your progress seems slow at first.

Exercise is the manifestation of what you do with your body. It's time to look at what you put into your body, to round out the great trifecta of treating Crohn's and autoimmune disease naturally.

Chapter Six

FOOD *DOES* MATTER

"The doctor of the future will give no medicine, but will instruct his patient in the care of the human frame, in diet and in the cause and prevention of disease."

—THOMAS EDISON

One of the most adamant lies told and repeated throughout my experience was that food plays no role in Crohn's disease. Consider for just a moment the reasoning behind that belief. Conventional doctors have told me that food plays no role, has zero impact on the health and well-being of a person's gastrointestinal tract. Food, allegedly, plays no role in how your mouth, throat, stomach, and intestines feel or function. The only equally insane analogy I can imagine would be if biologists claimed that the health of a fish has nothing to do with the water it lives in. It's absurd.

Food *does* matter, but what does this mean precisely? The food you eat determines your total body health. Ultimately, you have no choice but to eat. Eating is one of the four pillars of survival for all humans: food, water, air, and shelter. You do, however, have to choose what to eat, when to eat, and how much to eat. These decisions will shape your health at the cellular level, and manifest themselves in a variety of ways including in your skin, hair, mood, and muscle. Unfortunately, the Standard American Diet (SAD) is loaded with sugar, seed oils, and refined grains. This means that the default eating habits of many Americans are detrimental to their health. SAD foods are highly inflammatory and can trigger a natural propensity you may have to get an autoimmune disease.

In fact, the Standard American Diet may also be the primary driver behind the explosion in autoimmune diseases, including Crohn's. It is packed with processed flour, which has become increasingly dangerous to our health. In 2006, the herbicide glyphosate was approved in the US for spraying on wheat. Glyphosate is the active ingredient in Roundup, and since its introduction, the American population has experienced an explosion in autoimmune diseases, including celiac.[57] A 2013 paper found glyphosate to be a major cause of the increase in celiac disease—which is associated with other pathologies such as low iron and overgrowth of pathogens in the gut.[58] While science may still be debating the specific causes of these conditions, use your common sense. More Americans are chronically sick now than ever before. A lot has changed about the country over the last 250 years, including our environment and economy. But probably the most pertinent variable to a person's health is the food they eat. How our food is made is among the most profound changes. How could the two factors not be linked?

TRUST YOURSELF

Food is also one of the most intuitive aspects of health, along with exercise. That is, *you know* it works. You know you feel worse after eating junk food and doing nothing. You feel markedly better when you eat fresh fruit and go for a walk. There may not be official medical studies proving this, but then again, medical and scientific studies are often not done on the most obvious aspects of life. You don't need me to tell you that you will feel better after eating healthier and moving more—yet this view lacks credibility in circles where credentials are everything.

My doctors dismissed out of hand the possibility of using food as medicine shortly after my diagnosis. Their reasoning? The use of food and alternative diets to treat Crohn's hasn't been studied. The logic is laughable. *Try nothing that hasn't been done before.* Human civilization would still be progressing at a snail's pace if we were all required to advance under this guideline. Even when nutritionists are employed by your doctor to help address symptoms, they always seem to be placed on the back burner—a largely insignificant ordeal.

While I was still with the children's hospital, my doctor did have a staff nutritionist talk to me after my regular appointment. I tried not to laugh as she walked in. She was an older lady, no taller than five feet three inches, and very overweight. She talked for thirty minutes about Ritz crackers and milk being healthy snack options, among other things. When she finally left, I told my mother, "You've got to admit that was a waste of time." After transitioning to the adult doctor, I finally saw another dietitian. Skinny and fit, she instantly conveyed credibility. *Now that's a nutritionist*, I thought. Yet in four-and-a-half years with that doctor, I had only one appointment with the nutritionist. Never was there any mention about how diet could possibly replace my medication.

When treating Crohn's and other autoimmune diseases, there comes a point when you have to trust yourself (hopefully you're picking up on that!). Learning to trust your own judgment and intuition can save your life. Suggesting that food matters for your health may not seem like a groundbreaking concept, yet you would be surprised at the number of people still caught in the Big Healthcare trap that ignores nutrition.

Part of the problem is that Americans have become such unhealthy eaters that our perception of what healthy eating looks like has changed. Consider pre-industrial America once again. Those people ate only what they could grow, find, or kill. Of course, there were occasional opportunities to buy commodities such as sugar and salt for cooking, but these additives were not readily available. They were *occasional* treats, while the default eating habits remained healthy. Today, the opposite is true. The default eating habits now are unhealthy, ultra-processed snack foods. We come home and have food readily available in the refrigerator and cabinets. Grabbing food and eating it has never been easier, but this convenience comes with a cost to your health.

Many of you likely grew up eating what you thought was a fairly healthy diet. You always knew that a turkey sandwich, potato chips, and a chocolate chip cookie weren't as healthy as a broccoli and spinach salad. But it wasn't *that* bad either. We all seem to subconsciously think that stores would not be allowed to sell foods that could harm our health. It seemed reasonable to indulge in certain foods at times, or even on a regular basis.

Only now are many Americans beginning to realize that the foods they love are detrimental to their health and indeed can trigger the very autoimmune diseases we seek to cure. The problem with the SAD is that these foods may be okay for your body in moderation, but after repeated, regular consumption, your body becomes worn down metabolically by the chemicals, toxins, sugar, preservatives, and more in these products.

KNOW WHAT YOU CAN TOLERATE

There is so much nuance to treating Crohn's naturally. This means that your diet may not look like mine or someone else's. Dairy and eggs are especially contentious. Some w tolerate milk and yogurt with ease, while others vomit upon consuming them. Milk and cheese never sat well with me, even when I was little. Adding butter to any food has been eliminated from my supper plate as well. However, it is almost unavoidable to come across baked goods or any prepared dish with milk, butter, or cheese in it. Be your own judge. Sometimes small increments of these foods won't bother you, especially if they are consumed in addition to your "go-to" safe foods.

I highly recommend everyone keep a food diary—whether they have been diagnosed or not—with what they eat, when they eat, and the corresponding bowel movements they experience. You won't know what foods bother you unless you begin to keep track of what you are putting in your mouth. Once you start doing so, you will notice trends and quickly identify areas for improvement. It also helps keep you disciplined in the kitchen. You don't want to flip through your food diary and read repeated entries for chocolate cake and french fries.

It becomes a great way to track your diet and fitness routine, to mark your progress, and to note how you feel and if anything seems wrong. Keep up with how you feel after certain foods and workouts. If you ever find yourself in a funk for more than a few days, check your food journal and see what you were doing on the days you felt great. I have found this to be the best way to get back on track during lulls in my diet and fitness regimen.

I began keeping a food log shortly after coming home from my initial hospitalization and have continued to do so since. A majority of processed, fried, and sugary foods were instantly purged from my diet. The connection between these foods and decreases in my well-being was too obvious to ignore.

In addition to tracking the specific foods, track the time, place, circumstances, and how you are eating. Did you feel bad afterward because of the food itself or because of the environment you were in? Practice mindful eating. This means staying off your phone while you enjoy, and I mean truly *enjoy*, what you are eating. Chew your food into a thousand pieces before swallowing. Okay, maybe not that many. But don't be a steam shovel either. Chewing your food thoroughly has many digestive benefits. As you chew, your stomach activates digestive enzymes. When you chew your food into smaller pieces, stomach enzymes are better able to chemically break down your food and prepare it for absorption.

One irony of IBS is that inflammation can create such agony in the gut with its swollen intestines that certain processed foods are all that you can tolerate. The elemental diet (which will be discussed in a moment) is always your best bet while in the midst of a flare. However, if you don't have access to these products, you may resort to the healthiest version of processed food you can find. Look for crackers, bread, or pretzels with as few ingredients as possible, and chew them into mush—drink your solids—before swallowing. Again, this should just be a temporary solution until you can obtain some elemental diet formula.

How do you shop for healthy food when there is so much junk being sold in grocery stores? If you are going to chain grocery stores, you have to be a snob. Be picky and find the food that's good enough for you and your family. One old adage is to shop around the edges of any grocery store—where the fresh produce and meat are located. You may drift into the interior to find certain ingredients, such as organic nuts or dried fruit.

For those with IBD, I find it helpful to keep a list of your approved foods sold at each grocery store you shop at. You will be less tempted to deviate from the foods you know are good for you and don't trigger symptoms. It can be confusing for those who are just beginning to notice labels and are starting to be more mindful when they shop. You can easily be fooled. It's beyond the scope of this book to give a thorough breakdown. For a start, look out for added sugars, preservatives, natural flavors, food dyes, and ingredients you cannot pronounce. Avoid these when possible, or at least minimize your consumption.

INCREASING OPTIONS

A recent paper published in *Nutrients* captures the growing interest in using diet to treat Crohn's disease. The authors readily acknowledged that nutrition has always played a secondary role in Crohn's and noted the increasing prevalence of this autoimmune disease worldwide, among adults and children. Environmental factors such as antibiotic exposure during childhood, smoking exposure or addiction, and the modern Western diet itself are all, as the authors note, relevant factors and implicated in the early onset of Crohn's.[59]

We hear the term "Western diet" so often and know we are guilty of consuming it. It consists largely of white flour and sugar—ultra-processed food void of nutrients. But why, precisely, is our modern diet so harmful, and why does it have such a propensity to provoke autoimmune diseases such as Crohn's? You've probably heard of omega-3 fatty acids and omega-6 fatty acids in nutritional and health lexicons. Both have their place, and a healthy diet includes consuming omega-6 and omega-3 oils in a 1:1 to 4:1 ratio. However, our modern diet is now stacked heavily toward omega-6 fatty acids. It's estimated that the new ratio of consumption is 10:1 and as high as 20:1.[60] Omega-6 fatty acids are a source of inflammation and have gradually come to dominate the American diet as vegetable and seed oils have become prevalent in our food.

There are several factors that contribute to malnutrition and nutrient deficiency, which affect some 65–75 percent of all Crohn's patients.[61] Among the causes are poor absorption, small bacterial overgrowth, and loss of appetite. Fortunately, there are dietary alternatives to help you and others fight inflammation and autoimmune disease.

To start, there are some solid dietary approaches that Crohn's patients can implement, again depending on their unique symptoms. The Specific Carbohydrate Diet (SCD) was originally developed in the 1920s to treat celiac patients and was adopted in the early 1950s by a gastroenterologist to treat inflammatory bowel disease.[62] A case study is presented in just a few pages on a twenty-five-year-old who used this diet to treat Crohn's. The banned foods from this diet include: sucrose, maltose, isomaltose, lactose, potatoes, okra, corn, fluid milk, soy, cheese, food additives, and preservatives. Permitted foods include meat, eggs, oil, vegetables rich in amylose, nuts, and fruits. In children, this diet "promotes the mucosa healing" and "induces the normalization of inflammatory markers."[63]

Secondly, there is the low FODMAP diet, an acronym that stands for fermentable, oligosaccharides, disaccharides, mono-saccharides, and polyols. These collectively are the "banned" foods. They represent foods that are poorly absorbed and promote many of the symptoms associated with IBD including diarrhea, bloating, and abdominal pain. I have personal experience with this diet from working with my first functional medicine provider, and I enjoyed great success my first time around. It doesn't have to be perfect. There may be foods from the list of omitted foods that you tolerate perfectly fine. But following these guidelines, 80–90 percent worked wonders for me, in addition to supplements I was taking.

Another dietary option that has helped Crohn's patients is the semi-vegetarian diet. This diet does not omit meat and fish altogether, but they are limited. In addition to promoting overall gut health, one two-year study found that this diet helped prevent Crohn's patients in remission from experiencing any relapses.[64]

A 2021 paper published by Johns Hopkins University stated that "diet has shown some promise as a treatment alternative or accompaniment. The gut microbiome and diet are intrinsically linked to the emergence of IBD." The paper goes on to state, "New research has also shown associations between various foods and inflammation. Mediterranean diets, which are rich in monounsaturated fats, fiber, and omega-3 fatty acids, for example, have been associated with a significantly lower risk of later-onset CD [Crohn's disease]."[65] Meanwhile, foods like refined grains, saturated fats, glycemic carbohydrates, and high-energy soft drinks are associated with an increased risk of Crohn's.[66]

Again, it is worth remembering the nuance that comes with naturally treating Crohn's disease. While the Mediterranean diet may work for you, it may trigger symptoms in others. I know personally that olive oil, on the Mount Rushmore of health foods according to many, has not been good for my gut, and it's something I completely avoid. There is a mystery as to why certain foods cause symptoms and why others don't. Numerous physiological factors are at play, and no two people are identical.

Some people define remission or the complete state of healing as the point where you can truly eat anything you want and be asymptomatic. I strongly disagree with this approach. Even if you can drink Cokes and eat fries without incident, that doesn't mean you should consume them. My belief is the "as healthy as possible" approach. For instance, several food categories are permanently banned for me—like ice cream and alcohol. Other foods, like homemade bread at Christmas, may be consumed once a year on that special occasion without incident, but they are not something you make a permanent part of your life and diet.

Other diets, including the Paleolithic (paleo) diet, the Maker's Diet, and a vegan diet, may lack official approval in scientific circles and the medical establishment. I won't provide details on all of these, but Dr. Jordan Rubin has produced tremendous work with his book *Patient Heal Thyself*, in which he discusses The Maker's Diet, an invaluable guideline for me as I worked to harness the power of food. There are variations with all of these diets, but the overall theme remains the same: Eat whole, organic, natural foods. The nuance comes when considering your unique symptoms, and which healthy foods you may want to avoid until your gut is healed.

SUPPLEMENTS

Health supplements are all the rage. You may have seen probiotics and vitamins advertised on television, almost with the appeal of a miracle drug. Supplements, including vitamins and probiotics, are crucial weapons to combat autoimmune disease. This book is not, however, a medical encyclopedia, and not every probiotic, vitamin, and mineral can be listed with its benefits. There are literally thousands of supplements out there, and most of them are garbage. A few hundred are actually worthwhile, and they may not even be necessary for you and your condition.

Discovering what products I needed to add to my routine was essential to becoming drug-free, and I want you to do the same. Often this comes with having independent blood work and allowing a functional medicine provider or functional nutritionist to review your results and formulate a tailored plan for you. Still, there is so much you can learn on your own. Help from others is always great, but why not become your own expert too?

A 2022 paper published in *Foods* assessed the benefits of nutraceuticals and dietary supplements in the treatment of Crohn's disease. Nutraceuticals are foods that possess health-promoting properties, some of which can help treat Crohn's due to their anti-inflammatory properties. Moreover, they tend to be tolerated easily, as well as affordable and readily available. A broad range of products falls under this term, including herbal extracts, vitamins, peptides, and other micronutrients, along with dietary supplements such as probiotics.[67]

You may be taking various supplements and products right now, in addition to your official medical treatment. If you're like me, you discovered them on your own. There was always a very indifferent approach to these products by my GI doctors, and perhaps you have experienced these sentiments as well. Even the paper in *Foods* admits that "Clinicians often have a dismissive approach on the topic."[68] A major reason why you ventured into alternative treatments is because your pharmaceuticals are still leaving you with stubborn symptoms you cannot get rid of. By official medical standards, a patient may achieve remission, but many "IBD patients often suffer from overlapping functional irritable bowel syndrome-like (IBS-like) symptoms, such as bloating, abdominal pain and altered bowel frequency (diarrhea and/or constipation), which importantly affect their quality of life."[69] Hence the need to supplement, and hopefully replace altogether, your pharmaceuticals with the proper diet and exercise.

But what products and supplements should you take? It depends, because treating Crohn's and autoimmune disease naturally is based on each individual's unique needs. This is where it becomes very important to have independent blood testing for vitamin deficiencies, and then work with a functional medicine provider or functional nutritionist to create a healing strategy that works for you.

The paper in *Foods* made interesting observations about some specific supplements. Among the micronutrients that can help patients, "vitamin D and zinc play a relevant role in the immune system functioning and their deficiency has been linked to infectious and autoimmune disease, including CD."[70] The authors highlight the importance of zinc, adding that "Zinc is an essential micronutrient absorbed in the small intestine that appears to have anti-inflammatory and antioxidative properties."[71] Those with IBD who also suffer from zinc deficiency are more likely to end up in the hospital as well. Finally, polyunsaturated fats, which are abundant in fish oil, have anti-inflammatory properties.[72] Crohn's and most autoimmune diseases, even cancer, can be traced to inflammation. It's at the heart of so many health problems, so going natural requires an active approach to lowering your inflammation biomarkers.

When it comes to supplements, I cannot make blind recommendations without knowing your full health history. For me, it was game changing when I finally learned which ones to take based on my own blood tests in order to reduce inflammation and alleviate my symptoms. These included anti-inflammatories like fish oil and curcumin.

THE ELEMENTAL DIET

Many with Crohn's, IBD, or other autoimmune conditions may be so sick that they are unable to tolerate many healthy foods, including fruits and vegetables. While sick and in the midst of a flare, it is important to first get well. One approach involves a liquid diet, or elemental diet, which can work wonders. In fact, once I achieved remission, I continued to follow the elemental diet if symptoms suddenly reappeared. Even in the absence of symptoms, I usually consume a liquid-only meal at least once a day and periodically will go a full day with a liquid-only diet.

Enteral nutrition, or elemental diet formulas, are all-liquid approaches to consuming your calories, enabling your gut to rest and reset. Harmful gut bacteria, including *Bacteroidetes* species, are reduced or starved out. The exciting news about the elemental diet for younger patients (children and adolescents) is that it helps them achieve remission in about 75–85 percent of cases, and they are then able to reduce or end their use of steroids (which negatively affect their growth!).[73] How, specifically, does the elemental diet, or exclusive enteral nutrition (EEN) treatment, help patients? One of its many benefits is killing off, or rather starving out, bad bacteria. Certain bacteria in the gut, including *Bacteroides fragilis*, which can trigger symptoms and bad breath, feed on the conventional food we eat.

It also "promotes a reduction in the fecal calprotectin levels, a marker of gut inflammation; however, this effect is rapidly lost after food re-introduction."[74] This reason, among others, is why the elemental diet remains a consistent part of my routine—add the foods you can tolerate, but don't quit on this powerful supplement. Finally, this encouraging note is added about the benefits of the elemental diet: "After two weeks of treatment, patients treated with the oral elemental diet achieved the same clinical and laboratory remission as patients treated with corticosteroids, thus proving that an oral elemental diet could be as effective as steroids in inducing CD remission in adults."[75] That's good news for you and me.

Even some of the medical literature is starting to concede what should be obvious—that when it comes to treating Crohn's, food definitely matters. A 2024 article published in *Digestive Diseases and Sciences* reviewed the efficacy of the elemental diet. This protocol has been used for more than fifty years to treat a variety of diseases; however, elemental diets are often underutilized "due to poor palatability, access, cost, and lack of awareness regarding their clinical efficacy."[76] Elemental diets are a great option for so many reasons. They contain no food additives, are easily absorbed, help improve mucosal lining in the gut, and are allergen-free. Moreover, the liquid elemental diet generates little fecal bulk or buildup, granting relief for those with IBD suffering from diarrhea. Elemental diets consist of free amino acids and are a complete nutritional source—containing a daily requirement of vitamins and minerals.[77]

Knowledge is growing about the wonders of the elemental diet and its effectiveness in treating so many autoimmune diseases, including "inflammatory bowel diseases, small intestinal bacterial overgrowth...and celiac disease."[78] This article has a positive conclusion in regard to Crohn's, saying, "Overall, [the elemental diet] appears to be highly effective in inducing remission in adult and pediatric CD."[79] The authors have great news for kids and teenagers battling Crohn's, writing that "In children and adolescents, EEN [exclusive enteral nutrition] is recommended as first-line therapy for induction of remission."[80] The great benefit of treating yourself with a diet, including incorporating the elemental diet into your routine, is that there are virtually no side effects. What a relief compared to the dangerous pharmaceuticals!

An article published in *Nutrients* presented the results of a 12-week study involving 144 patients with Crohn's disease. These patients were treated with a semi-elemental diet, which resulted in improved nutritional status. Other symptoms improved across the board as well. "The mean number of stools per day significantly decreased," as the average number of bowel movements decreased from 4.6 per day to 1.7 per day at the end of the 12-week nutritional support program.[81] For those with IBD and IBS, we know what a relief that is. Just as important as treating symptoms, the authors wrote, "One of the most important findings of the study is the significant improvement in disease activity after 12 weeks of nutritional treatment."[82]

When you are experiencing symptoms, the elemental diet is your best bet at resolving the issues—beyond addressing stress or other factors that may have triggered your relapse of symptoms in the first place.

SUCCESS CASES

The Johns Hopkins paper mentioned earlier provided a case study of a twenty-five-year-old man who suffered from IBD and was initially on infliximab, a biologic that he soon developed antibodies to. After years of conventional treatment, he experienced a relapse of symptoms. Then he adhered to the elemental diet for two weeks. This was followed by a modified elemental diet in which half his calories came from food. The results: His fecal calprotectin, a marker of gastrointestinal inflammation, dropped from 453.5 to 65 in just five months. After the elemental diet, he transitioned to an exclusion diet that omitted grains, processed foods, alcohol, dairy, and eggs.[83]

The elemental diet worked wonders for this young man, and

it has for me as well. As an added source of encouragement, this patient continued to have success on the exclusion diet, which required him to cook all of his food, including fruits and vegetables. This increased his fiber intake and proved beneficial as "dietary fiber has been shown to inhibit inflammation."[84]

A second case study I want to highlight involves a twelve-year-old boy who was diagnosed with Crohn's disease.[85] Crohn's disease is more prevalent among children than ever before, and the dangers of being placed on pharmaceuticals at an early age pose a great risk. Those with young children at risk, or already diagnosed, should take notice. As we'll see, through the power of nutrition, it is possible to kill the bear in its den and avoid a lifetime of dependency on Big Pharma.

This boy was experiencing all the typical symptoms of IBD, including chronic diarrhea, intermittent fever, and abdominal pain. As if on cue, a colonoscopy was performed, and he was diagnosed with Crohn's and placed on omeprazole (brand name Prilosec)—a conventional Big Pharma treatment.[86] (Again, the absurdity of pharmaceuticals needs to be highlighted. Among its many side effects, omeprazole causes diarrhea and stomach pain—the very symptoms this young boy was experiencing in the first place!)[87] After over ten months of this and other treatments, his symptoms were not improving. They were, in fact, getting worse, as rectal bleeding occurred. Dietary measures were tried next. The patient was placed on the Lifestyle Eating and Performance (LEAP) program. The LEAP program is "an elimination diet built on the selection of less-immunoreactive foods and chemicals" identified by test results.[88]

This patient was also "placed on an anti-yeast protocol (no added sugar, vinegar, mushrooms, peanuts, or pistachios, and fruits were limited to two servings [per day])."[89] His LEAP program consisted of "about 40 least-immune-reactive foods in a nutritionally balanced manner," all arranged by his dietitian.[90] After the first two weeks, other foods were gradually reincorporated into his diet. In addition to these dietary guidelines, he took a series of supplements including: Curcumax Pro, antifungals, grapefruit seed extract, garlic extract, and probiotics including *Saccharomyces boulardii*.[91]

The results were extraordinary. After just thirty-nine days, his calprotectin decreased dramatically—by over 90 percent. After four months on this elimination diet, "there was a remarkable remission of symptoms with no abdominal pain complaints."[92] Hallelujah! The loose bowel movements were gone and so, too, was the rectal bleeding. There were noticeable gains in his weight and height, and he was able to reduce his use of supplements. After one year on the LEAP program, a "colonoscopy showed normal visible and histologic findings with 10 biopsies from the esophagus to the sigmoid colon."[93] Just a few months later, the patient "reported no abdominal pain, diarrhea, or other gastrointestinal symptoms and had an estimated healthy weight and height for his age."[94] Over three years later, he was still in clinical remission and enjoyed normal growth and healthy weight gain for his age. He continued to avoid processed foods and food chemicals. Best of all, he remained drug-free.[95]

These cases demonstrate once again that it can be done. You can come off your biologics, or whatever pharmaceutical drug you are bound to, and utilize the great healing power of food. The comfort that comes from allowing real, whole foods into your body, and knowing they will treat and cure you, while avoiding dangerous pharma products, is unmatched. Why is diet not used more often? Why do doctors persist in prescribing drugs when actual healing can be achieved by harnessing proper nutrition? It would take another book to fully address, but part of the answer is financial. To heal yourself by eating well, along with exercise and strong faith, means you can no longer be a pincushion for the nurses in the infusion center and lab center. There's no need for constant appointments. There is far less money to be made from a healthy patient. Another major reason is lack of awareness; people simply don't know how to—or don't have the self-confidence to—tell their doctor they want to try something else. I hope to change that.

If you don't know where to begin, start with the basics I have outlined. Depending on the severity of your case, some of you will be able to take the appropriate steps on your own to cure Crohn's, IBD, or any condition you struggle with. For many, an experienced functional nutritionist or functional medicine provider can help you tailor your diet so you can harness the power of food to finally cure your autoimmune disease.

Chapter Seven

TAKE CHARGE

"Do what you can, with what you have, where you are."
—THEODORE ROOSEVELT

The country may be in the early stages of a national health revolution, but don't wait for policymakers to improve your health. Take the initiative and act now. Besides, now you've got the triad of factors necessary for self-healing—faith, fitness, and nutrition. It's time to put it all together. I truly believe that healing yourself naturally will work as you apply these basic principles, but it goes beyond what I have outlined. It is important to return to the root causes of IBD and identify factors that may have been a contributing factor in your diagnosis—and factors that may continue to prolong your symptoms.

Those of us in the natural healing and clean living space know there are so many factors to consider. It's up to you to decide how thorough you want to be with your healing and health. Research has shown that your dental health may be a contributing factor in autoimmune diseases. Mercury amalgam fillings in your teeth, and other heavy metal exposure, are a possible contributing factor to autoimmune disease, including IBD and IBS.[96] Even your cookware needs to be considered, as chemicals, toxins, and metals in these materials can be harmful as well.[97] Reduce plastics as much as possible—including bags, bottles, and other containers. These plastics contain chemicals such as xenoestrogens, which can wreck your immune system.[98] There is a lot to consider!

If you have an autoimmune disease, it's up to you to take action if you want to be well. Start your fitness routine. Start eating healthier. If you don't yet have one, start a relationship with God and ask Him to heal you.

Imagine the healthy life you want to have. A life with no symptoms, no pharmaceuticals, no doctor's appointments, no tests, and no more insecurity or stigma caused by the disease you once carried. Have a clear vision of where you want to take your health, and imagine how good it will feel to finally get there. But in order to make this a reality, you must *choose* to be healthy. Decide that being sick isn't an option and that you will relentlessly pursue the goal of becoming the healthiest version of yourself. Can you become healthy just by will? I believe so.

I assure you that your body will respond to what you tell yourself. A poor mindset becomes a self-fulfilling prophecy. Tell yourself you'll be sick, and you most likely will be. Decide to be healthy, and you are well on your way to a much more fulfilling life.

If you want to overcome Crohn's, ulcerative colitis, or any autoimmune disease, the first step is to make the decision to do so. I know for me the true moment of healing began when I believed in my heart and gut that I could come off my biologics and be perfectly fine—in fact, better than fine. It may take decades for America's health revolution to produce public policy that helps people become healthier by default—that is, before all the bad food in the grocery store is removed, before harmful vaccines are stopped, and before other absurd medical practices that are routine in American clinics are stopped. Until this happens, you must choose to be healthy.

LOG YOUR SYMPTOMS

Time is a scarce resource. Not everything can be done or fixed in a day. So, we rank items. We prioritize certain tasks over others based on our own individual preferences. During a household fire, for instance, everyone would grab the children rather than slowly poke around for trinkets as the flames burn.

Thomas Sowell, one of my favorite economists, gives a great example of an army medic with limited supplies who's confronted with three wounded soldiers. One soldier is likely to live regardless of whether his injuries are treated. A second soldier is so badly hurt that only a team of doctors with a high-tech operating room could save his life. A third soldier may be wounded, but will surely die if his ailments are not addressed. However, this third soldier's injuries are less severe than the second soldier's. Therefore, if the army medic can save only one, he will use the few supplies he has to save the third soldier.

Your healing process should function in a similar way. For many with IBD or IBS, the most urgent need will be to control stomach pain. I personally know how bad this symptom can get, and it is clear why this one should be tackled first. Other symptoms of preeminent importance may include diarrhea, rectal bleeding, fistula, poor appetite and/or absorption, as well as body aches and pains. Some symptoms, such as acne, are top of mind to heal as well, but perhaps not as urgent as having diarrhea twenty-plus times a day. Moreover, the beauty of treating Crohn's and autoimmune disease naturally is that taking steps to address one symptom may help clear up others as well—an added bonus even if you didn't intend to treat it first. For example, say a patient stops eating sugar to help with their stomach pain and notices that their acne has disappeared in the process. It's a win-win!

I've already mentioned the importance of keeping a daily log or journal of what you eat. It's a good idea whether you have an autoimmune disease or not. You might as well keep a big journal. Record your workouts, diet, symptoms, weight, etc., all in one place each day. This is the only way to start detecting patterns in your diet and lifestyle so you can make changes accordingly. You need to write down and rank your symptoms as they occur, from urgent to mild. You'll soon have volumes of notebooks recording your daily habits and dietary intake. It becomes a treasure trove of information for you and your body. Over time, you will notice patterns that will let you take charge of your healing.

In the course of making your daily notes and entries, patterns will present themselves. Clear distinctions will be made regarding the food you eat and how you feel afterward. Now, list your symptoms—even if you have some that you believe are unrelated to your official diagnosis. The body is a complex, interconnected system. Everything is related in some manner. For instance, say a patient has the following symptoms and ranks them as follows:

SYMPTOMS

- Stomach pain
- Nausea
- Diarrhea
- Headache

The next step is to focus efforts on tackling each symptom from the top down. You may find that one symptom is easy to conquer. For instance, stomach pain was my number one symptom during at least five major flare-ups. In the course of your experience, you will quickly learn which foods to avoid. That is, those foods that trigger inflammation in your intestines. You will also learn that stress and environmental factors can cause symptoms, including stomach pain.

Once you recognize these, develop mechanisms for handling situations differently, or avoiding them altogether. For example, men who are passionate about football or baseball may get so worked up over a game, that those with IBD or IBS start feeling symptoms. A passionate attachment to sports can have other harmful effects on men's health as well, such as a drop in testosterone when your team loses.[99] I love sports as much as anyone, but I had to learn how to detach myself emotionally from the outcome. The same can be true of politics, hunting, a building project, or anything that could be frustrating if it doesn't go your way. Curing autoimmune disease naturally comes with lifestyle changes, and while I don't think you need to give up anything you enjoy (that may be detrimental) you do need to take an honest look at how some of your habits, routines, hobbies, and interests—or lack thereof—may either be helping or hurting your health.

ASSESS SYMPTOM RELAPSES

It requires vigilance to remain symptom-free when dealing with Crohn's. You have to constantly listen to your gut.

Even after becoming drug-free, you may notice that symptoms will reappear. They did for me at times and still occasionally reappear. Part of it is you're human, and no human body functions perfectly all the time. It's important not to panic; instead, remain calm. Breathe and pray your way out of any bad spell. Praise God and Jesus when the symptoms subside and reflect on what went wrong that led to this sudden relapse; I can't stress this enough. I mentioned in Chapter 3 how my innate aversion to going to the doctor made my experience all the more ironic. Aside from my major hospitalizations, I tried to avoid the hospital and developed a high tolerance for pain. I'm not by any means suggesting you should suffer through unbearable pain. During my 2018 spell, I desperately needed pain medication and am grateful it was administered. But at other times, for me (and for men in general) there's nothing wrong with learning how to handle pain—learning to calm yourself and make yourself comfortable until it passes. If you are working with a functional medicine provider or functional nutritionist, let them know about symptoms that come up again.

When symptoms reappear for me, I immediately prescribe myself an elemental diet and a fast from solid foods, along with time outdoors when possible. Fortunately, by the time you achieve the drug-free state of treating IBD, you'll likely have years' worth of notebooks detailing your food during that time, in addition to how you felt. There are several factors that can cause a relapse of symptoms. You may have been mad about something or someone. Maybe you have not exercised due to a busy schedule or injury. You may have pushed the boundaries of your dietary restrictions—or eaten while you were stressed or angry. In short, I have noticed that falling out of routine can trigger symptoms.

For instance, your sleep schedule may be thrown off because of travel, work, or stress. It could be that you ran low on the foods you regularly consume and had to temporarily dip into food groups that are normally forbidden based on your needs.

In the old days when my symptoms reappeared, I would call my doctor, who would immediately prescribe medicine and order tests and blood work. None of it ever did any good, as I always ended up fixing myself on my own—either by waiting out the painful spell or tweaking my diet as needed to extinguish the symptoms that reappeared.

Travel is not always bad for your health. In fact, a trip to the beach has worked wonders for my health and that of many others. The sun seems to have healing powers as it shines on your stomach; in the same way, it can disinfect anything else left to its exposure. There is typically unwarranted pressure to always be doing something on vacation. Take time to relax, meditate, and pray on the beach. Isolate yourself for a time and close your eyes while you listen to waves reach the shore. If you can't make the beach, I have found that being outdoors in general, or nature therapy, has tremendous therapeutic and healing powers. If you find yourself in an urban environment, escape the stress, crowds, noise, and pollution and enjoy a few days, or even just a few hours, in the country—whether it's a park or your favorite getaway. Sometimes just a few hours to stare at the trees, the mountains, or the ocean is enough to reenergize and rejuvenate. Keep track of how your stomach feels and how your symptoms are doing before and after any getaway. Of course, if they improve, try to make the outdoor retreat a consistent part of your life if it isn't already.

The importance of exercise and nutrition has already been covered in previous chapters, so I won't rehash these points. In continuing to stay drug-free, there is an important comparison to note about curing autoimmune disease and your fitness routine.

Think about your gut health like training in the gym. You could spend a year training, weight lifting, and building the physique of your dreams. If you sculpt your body—through diet and exercise—into something you're proud of, can you expect to maintain peak physical shape without some effort? Of course not! Yes, you've done the hard work of getting your body to where you want to be, but now you have to continue to train and follow the proper diet if you want the results to last. I want your good health to last too, which is why you have to stay vigilant. It may take a few weeks, a few months, or a year of discipline to finally heal yourself naturally. Once you do, most of your eating and daily habits should remain in place. You'll be so grateful to be symptom-free that you most likely won't miss the foods you used to eat. Even if cravings linger, remember this: The guy in the gym who has already built his body could skip a workout or have a cheat meal with little effect on his overall health. Similarly, after you have put in the work to finally overcome Crohn's and other autoimmune diseases, there will be times when you can indulge in your favorite foods without triggering symptoms.

Some of you may prefer to have a functional health provider or a nutritionist help you every step of the way. There's nothing wrong with that! For others, you may refer to specialists on an as-needed basis when symptoms suddenly reappear and you are struggling to resolve them.

INVEST IN YOUR HEALTH

If you are fed up with your current doctor or treatment plan and feel that the quality of your health has stagnated or declined for years, it's time to go all-in on being healthy and maximizing your time on earth. This requires investing in yourself. School-children and young adults are now targeted, in a good way, with information about the need to save and invest for retirement.

We are taught to have millions of dollars saved up for when we are old. That way, the logic goes, we can live comfortably in retirement. First, retirement is a flawed concept. This is a separate book, but once you find your purpose and passion in life, why ever stop? There are too many examples of widely successful and healthy people who stopped working and died a short time later. None of this is to pretend that death isn't real, or that you shouldn't build wealth for later in life. Of course, death is inevitable, and you need to be responsible about your future finances.

But it's far more important to take care of yourself now. What good is $10 million in thirty years if you don't live to spend it? Living healthy requires that you invest in your health. It means being willing to pay more for healthier food options, for independent blood testing, and for the services of a functional medicine doctor or functional nutritionist. We are willing to pay enormous sums for almost anything including homes, cars, phones, clothes, jewelry, vacations, boats, TVs, and so on. Your health deserves more attention than any of these things.

I grew up in my father's school of finance; his monetary habits defined what it meant to be fiscally responsible. He could squeeze 103 cents out of every dollar and used 1960s-era prices as his comparison point for all purchases. Thrift was a part of growing up. You just didn't spend money. Unfortunately, this otherwise sound financial advice proved detrimental to my health.

For years I avoided paying for a functional medicine provider, independent blood testing, or any supplements to account for my nutritional deficiencies. Only when I was at the end of my rope did I break down and make the necessary expenditures to finally get myself better. For many with autoimmune disease, you need to pay these expenses as necessary, depending on your unique symptoms and circumstances. Achieving a full recovery may even require you to move. If you are in an area with toxins, heavy metals, chemicals, mold, or odors that are triggering your symptoms, it may be worth the financial commitment to relocate to a fresh environment to focus on your health.

This is another regrettable mistake that I, and others, have made: delaying our own recovery. I made the mistake of putting off self-care and curing myself for good, foolishly thinking that at some point in the future it might be easier or more ideal. I used to think about curing myself naturally when I was in my late teens and early twenties. I frequently thought when I was nineteen or twenty that once I was married, and working, I'd finally be able to sit down and figure out how to cure myself naturally. If you're having these same thoughts, don't wait. You'll never be in a perfect position to do anything. This includes getting healthy, so act on it now. If you are delaying your own healing process because you think it will be easier once you're married, or have a certain job, or turn a certain age, understand that these future possibilities may not even be there if you don't act today and get your body healed.

Your health is worth investing in. Even if you can't afford to spend thousands of dollars on specialized providers or supplements, there are many free steps, or less expensive steps, you can take. The crucial mindset shift, which will be explained in a moment, is a great free first step, as is embracing Christianity and biblical teachings to help you through your journey. Investing in yourself costs nothing but a little time to start exercising at home. Going for a nice walk and doing a few bodyweight exercises are great ways to get started. Spending a few extra dollars at the grocery store or going to a farmers' market to buy healthier food is well worth it. Quality is worth paying for. If your symptoms are not severe, or at worst mild, these small changes alone could significantly reduce them or eliminate them altogether. What a blessing!

The best professional athletes spend an enormous amount of money on their bodies. They pay for the best physicians, trainers, chefs, therapy, and other treatments. They prioritize sleep and recovery. They each treat their body the way a racehorse is treated, the way you should treat yourself. Athletes prioritize their well-being and invest heavily in taking care of their bodies because it is the ultimate tool that allows them to perform and compete at a high level. It's how they get paid and earn a handsome living.

Your body is also worth investing in, and reinvesting in. We can't all be professional athletes, but we can all prioritize our health. Sure, you may never have the means to spend a million dollars annually on a personal trainer, chef, supplements, etc. But you can make small daily investments that pay off big time. You only have one body, so treat it well.

Healing didn't truly take effect for me until I moved, changed states and vocations, and headed further south. Before becoming drug-free, it seemed I would remain tethered to Vanderbilt for life as long as I stayed in Tennessee. I needed a way out and went back to school in another state, in large part to finally escape my doctors back home. Although I continued with my conventional treatments for several months thereafter, I had already started to dabble in functional medicine. Here's the rest of the story.

SHIFT YOUR MINDSET

For years I took a very passive approach to my health. Even when I felt fine, I believed my doctors at Vanderbilt when they said I was still sick. For too long, I just rolled with the punches my conventional doctors threw at me. As I approached my mid-twenties and was still sick, it dawned on me how abnormal this approach was. Young men are not supposed to be sick. We are supposed to be the healthiest people society has to offer. I was so tired of being told I was sick for life and internalizing this medical propaganda. This is why my mindset shift was so important.

Before discussing the crucial shift, I want to clarify that my outlook wasn't always negative. By now you understand how important fitness is to overcoming Crohn's. Even while I was still on biologic drugs, I still managed to have great workouts. I didn't lack enthusiasm in the gym. I always loved hitting the weights hard and having a great workout. My mindset was not in the gutter, but I knew there was something missing.

After years of being inundated with the "sick for life" dogma, I had internalized that outlook. It became a mental obstacle that I never realized I needed to overcome. For years, there were times when I felt 80–90 percent cured. But I never knew what the last piece was or how to get it. I wanted to come off of Remicade and ditch the doctor, but I lacked the gumption to act. As I began to research alternative treatment methods, and discover other people with Crohn's who cured themselves naturally, a new level of confidence developed. I ordered Jini Patel Thompson's book *Listen to Your Gut* and was already following many of the protocols included to help IBD patients. What's more, she described the maintenance diet to help Crohn's patients continue to live symptom-free. My diet seemed good enough to keep me healthy, and I was still exercising, but I was still having trouble. However, the more I researched and the more I kept exercising, the more I began to believe I could also take a different approach to healing.

In August 2023, I had my first appointment with a functional medicine provider in the United Kingdom, known as "The Gut Expert." We talked for an hour over Zoom, and I shared my health history. The amount of time she spent with me was unusual and a relief, compared to the short routine appointments I was used to at Vanderbilt. Her daughter had Crohn's disease, and a bad case of it. Yet she was able to cure herself naturally. I learned so much during this call, and it set the stage for future calls with other functional medicine providers. During our meeting, I told her I believed I could come off Remicade and be fine. This was not recommended by her (or my doctors), but I was encouraged by what she said afterward. I'll summarize her response: *Although I never recommend quitting cold turkey, keep this in mind. If you truly believe that you can come off Remicade and be fine, you are probably right. Remember, listen to your gut!*

It took about eight more months, more appointments, and more symptoms, before I finally took this leap of faith and quit Remicade. But I had built the mindset to do so. The final mental gear was in place. Not only was I fine-tuning my diet, continuing with an exercise regimen, and growing in my faith, but also the crucial link was now there—an intense belief that I could cure myself naturally and become a healthier version of myself. And if that were possible, if I could come off Remicade and be symptom-free, then I could also reject the conventional medical mindset of being "sick for life."

This mental shift was free and always there for the taking. I came to this realization the long way. I'm better off for it, but imagine if I had acted on it sooner. Imagine if you act on it today. Crohn's was not a lifelong burden. This disease gave me plenty of challenges, to be sure, but it was always within my capacity to overcome it.

I saw Crohn's not as a debilitating illness, but as a rite of passage to becoming a stronger and healthier version of myself. How do you see your diagnosis? I have come across online message boards where Crohn's patients take offense at the notion that you can heal yourself naturally. Maybe these people are lashing out because they are in the midst of a flare, and they have my sympathy if so. Still, you have to decide how optimistic you will remain about your body and health. You must choose to be healthy. Your body will respond to the things you tell it. Tell yourself you'll be sick, and you most likely will be. Decide to be healthy, and you are well on your way to a more fulfilling life.

I found tremendous confidence in my *good* days with Crohn's—those precious symptom-free days when I felt great and had tremendous workouts. I wanted that feeling all the time. I truly believed in my gut that I could come off of Remicade and thrive.

In order to become drug-free, you have to make that decision within yourself. Tell yourself positive things. *I know I can be healthy and thrive without the use of pharmaceuticals. In fact, I know I can be even healthier, and finally LIVE, L-I-V-E, after being held back by this supposedly incurable condition. I can finally achieve goals and aspirations that I put off for years because of this disease.*

You have to truly believe that you know your body better than anyone else. No doctor or physician understands your medical history better than you do. How could they? You know virtually every aspect of your health, how you feel, your energy, your diet, your weight, and a host of other factors. Any physician who only makes a few minutes for you, a few times a year, cannot possibly glean more information about you than you already know. Trust yourself! A functional nutritionist or functional medicine provider may be great to work with, and they can often provide far greater insights and spend more time with you than conventional doctors ever have.

Believe that you can overcome your autoimmune disease and health challenges. Believe that you can come off your pharmaceuticals and thrive. Believe that you can take charge of your health and unleash a new version of yourself. This was, in many ways, the key to me becoming drug-free with Crohn's disease. At many points over the years, I occasionally believed I could be fine without Remicade or my gastroenterologist. Yet it was only a half-hearted belief. When you make a commitment to yourself to go all-in on curing yourself naturally and are driven by a belief that you can indeed do it, then you will witness remarkable outcomes in your health and life.

Healing likely won't happen overnight. It may only take a few days or weeks for those with light or mild cases, but for others, it may take several months to a year. Although I was diagnosed at twelve, I was twenty-six before I finally figured out how to address the root causes of my condition. Becoming drug-free was the most liberating experience and allowed me the chance—for the first time—to truly live with confidence after I beat the insecurity Crohn's had caused for so long.

For years, doctors, hospitals, and Big Pharma felt like an albatross around my neck. I spent the best years of my youth living with a condition I was told was incurable. If you have as well, my advice to you is this: Learn from what's behind you but keep moving forward. Maybe there were missed opportunities in life because of your illness, and that's regrettable, but don't dwell on the years and time you believe were lost. The best thing to do is thank God for getting you this far and for giving you a chance to get healthy now. Be grateful for the second chance and resolve not to squander the opportunity to restore your health.

CONCLUSION

It was July 2024. I had been off Remicade for more than three months—longer than any period since 2011—and I was thriving. I couldn't believe how good I felt, and how the symptoms I always dealt with seemed to have disappeared. Part of me immediately wished that I had done this years ago. That is, firing my doctors and quitting my medicine. I did not dwell long on the regret of not having acted sooner. I was glad I finally did. I felt free to live for the first time. Free to travel. Free to move. Free to take risks. Free to go on dates. I want you to experience the same thing.

It was in July 2024 that I received a heavy calling on my heart to write this book. I have always been a private person, perhaps the most offline guy in my generation. I never had social media until recently. (Men are not supposed to be self-revealers, remember!) But I felt such a strong call to try and help others, and I started working on this book. It was slow going at first, but my efforts began in earnest in January 2025.

This book was a challenge, and there were plenty of frustrating moments over the course of several months. I kept thinking of the next twelve-year-old boy, somewhere across America, whose doctor has just diagnosed him with Crohn's disease. I want this book to reach him and his parents. Getting diagnosed with Crohn's is scary. The symptoms are dreadful, but I don't want anyone with Crohn's to have irreversible surgery or fall into the "sick for life" trap. It took me years to learn what I have shared with you, and I hope you apply these lessons and take agency over your own health.

Although I got my master's to work in public policy or academia, I knew I had to help others after healing myself. That's why I launched Drug-Free Crohn's to help you and anyone with autoimmune disease become the healthiest version of yourself. If you have Crohn's, colitis, or another autoimmune disease, I want to hear from you. Send me an email to drugfreecrohns@gmail.com. I'd love to connect with you, learn your story, and work with you in my independent health coaching practice.

YOUR NEXT STEPS

Remember that IBD can be triggered by stress, environmental factors, toxins, chemicals, and certain foods and beverages. Work to identify which of these in your home or work could be contributing to your symptoms, and try to eliminate or reduce them. I used to be prone to skin infections like impetigo and sinus infections. My doctor always recommended washing with antibacterial soap—which I dutifully did for years. It wasn't until I started learning about alternative healing protocols that I finally learned that antibiotics, including antibacterial soap, can trigger symptoms of IBD. I'm still learning too. The important thing is to just start gradually incorporating more and more protocols, practices, and insights into your daily health routine. Again, there is no one-size-fits-all approach to treating autoimmune disease. Listen to your body and take big leaps or incremental steps to improve your health as needed.

The trials presented by Crohn's and other autoimmune diseases offer one encouraging aspect: You and your body have been through so much. Looking back, you may feel anger or resentment for the years of being sick instead of healthy. But consider where you are today, now that you are drug-free and thriving. There is so much you have overcome. Be proud of yourself for finally conquering the greatest challenge in your life. More challenges in other areas lie ahead, but you now have something most people don't: You've been through the wringer and come out on the other side a stronger, healthier, more confident version of yourself. If life has another daunting task for you ahead, this time you'll be able to face it with a healthy, fit body—one that's far more capable of handling the next trial than the sickly version of yourself contending with the rigors of autoimmune disease.

After you beat autoimmune disease, so many opportunities open up, personally and professionally. Opportunities that you may have previously declined due to your illness are suddenly appealing and there for you. That happened for me—I rediscovered opportunities that would not have been possible in previous years, as thinking about my upcoming Remicade appointment or what to do if symptoms appeared would drown out my plans.

For nearly fifteen years, I let Crohn's hold me back. Now I am drug-free and truly living my best life. No matter what stage you are at in your health journey, it is never too late to take charge of your health. Perhaps you have no health challenges of your own. My hope is that you are in the active preventative stage, living the best you can and making lifestyle choices that will continue to promote your good health. For those still struggling, it is my fervent desire to see you become well. I pray you may have found some inspiration and hope in these words.

Although it is often difficult to navigate the storms life throws at you, including autoimmune disease, there is a much better life on the other side.

APPENDIX

There is so much more to talk about when it comes to conventional treatment for Crohn's, colitis, and autoimmune disease. I originally included all of the following medications with their side effects in Chapter 3. I realized after reading it what a bore this could be for the reader, and instead moved this material to an appendix. Here are some common pharmaceutical treatments prescribed by doctors to treat Crohn's disease, ulcerative colitis, and IBS. These details are taken from the medications' own websites and from the FDA. Here are the medications in addition to their common side effects:

PREDNISONE

When prednisone was first introduced on the marketplace in 1955, it came with instructions from the manufacturer that it was only to be used in "life-threatening situations."[100] It is now handed out to children liberally (I took prednisone as a child). As a steroid medication, one of the most visible side effects is the moon-face look.

Here are some of the other, many more serious side effects of Prednisone: difficulty sleeping, weight gain, acne, headache and dizziness, nausea and stomach pain.

RINVOQ (UPADACITINIB)

Rinvoq was approved by the FDA to treat UC and Crohn's disease in 2023 and works by suppressing the immune system.[101] From its own website, "RINVOQ is a Janus kinase (JAK) inhibitor that works inside your cells to block certain signals that are *thought* to cause inflammation" (emphasis added).[102] Medicine is still a practice, and there is no greater reminder than reviewing the literature provided by the drug makers themselves. There are few certainties and absolute truths. Much is still unknown, as this statement testifies to this old adage.

Major side effects include:

- Serious infections
- Increased risk of death in people over fifty with at least one heart disease risk factor
- Cancer and immune system problems, including lymphoma and lung cancer
- Increased risk of major cardiovascular events
- Blood clots
- Allergic reactions
- Tears in the stomach or intestines (You already have Crohn's or UC!)
- Changes in certain blood tests

These are all in addition to the myriad of common side effects including:

- Fever, sweating, or chills
- Shortness of breath
- Warm, red, or painful skin or sores
- Muscle aches
- Feeling tired
- Blood in phlegm
- Diarrhea or stomach pain
- Cough
- Weight loss
- Burning when urinating or increased frequency of urination

SKYRIZI

Skyrizi is another relatively new drug on the market, approved by the FDA in 2019.[103] Among the more alarming risks for Crohn's patients include hepatotoxicity, or liver damage, during administration of the drug.[104] From the website of the drug itself, here are the major side effects:

- Hypersensitivity reactions
- Infection
- Tuberculosis (TB)
- Hepatotoxicity in treatment of inflammatory bowel disease (Crohn's and colitis)
- Upper respiratory infections
- Headache
- Arthralgia in induction and arthralgia
- Abdominal pain
- Injection-site reaction
- Anemia
- Pyrexia
- Back pain

- Arthropathy
- Urinary tract infection (UTI)

It's not just drug websites where you can find shocking revelations about their products. A recent academic paper reviewed current treatments for Crohn's disease and acknowledged that "many IBD patients do not respond adequately to most biologics."[105]

Again, biologics refers to medications or medical treatments that use genetic material of living organisms in their production. If biologics have harmful side effects, and patients don't tolerate them well, why are we still using them? Why are biologic drugs often the first response by the doctors who receive a new IBD patient?

The current treatment options for IBD are not ideal; they only seek to achieve remission, not completely heal the body. Several medications and conventional treatments for IBD, Crohn's, and ulcerative colitis are discussed, including their side effects. Some of the key points are worth including here. The paper states that treatment for IBD initially relied on drugs like corticosteroids and immunosuppressants for many years.[106]

Today, common oral medications for ulcerative colitis include: olsalazine, balsalazide, and sulfasalazine. However, these medications "are associated with side effects, including cardio- and hepatorenal toxicity and sexual dysfunction."[107]

There are four primary corticosteroids used to treat Crohn's and colitis: budesonide, prednisone, hydrocortisone, and methylprednisone. All four have the same potential side effects, including: acne, weight gain, fragility, hypertension, diabetes, moon face, insomnia, mood swings, weakened bones (osteoporosis), and increased risk of infection.[108]

Azathioprine, 6-mercaptopurine, and tacrolimus are among

the immunosuppressants used to treat Crohn's and colitis. Aza-thioprine is used for patients with steroid-dependent diseases to delay the recurrence of Crohn's after surgical resection. It's an oral medication that can cause pancreatitis, suppression of bone marrow, and lymphoma.[109]

6-mercaptopurine is used in patients with steroid-resistant or steroid-dependent disease to delay the recurrence of CD after surgical resection, and can cause headaches, diarrhea, nausea, vomiting, tiredness, joint pain, mouth sores, fever, and liver inflammation.[110] Many of these side effects are symptoms of Crohn's, and other autoimmune diseases in general. Are patients expected to distinguish between diarrhea caused by IBD and diarrhea caused by the medication? This sounds like taking a pill to cure a headache, only the pill causes a headache too.

Tacrolimus, an oral medication for Crohn's disease, can cause diabetes, hepatitis, decreased kidney function, increased cholesterol, high blood pressure, headache, swollen gums, and seizures.[111] You could take this medication to "treat" Crohn's and get diabetes in the process. Anyone up for that?

TNF (tumor necrosis factor) inhibitors seek to work by blocking the inflammation induced by TNF in the first place.[112] One of these medications is adalimumab (Humira). Humira can cause injection-site reactions, headaches, nausea, abdominal pain, vomiting, upper respiratory infections (sinus infection), and muscle pain.[113]

A second is infliximab (Remicade, Inflectra, and others), which can be used for both Crohn's and colitis. These drugs can cause fever, chest pain, respiratory infections such as sinus infection, sore throat, sweating, nausea, itching, headache, coughing, rash, difficulty breathing, and stomach pain. Again, so many of these are symptoms of the disease itself.

This paper adds in regard to TNF inhibitors: "Although TNF inhibitors are one of the preferred therapies for IBD, their repeated use may induce immunogenicity."[114]

Janus kinase (JAK) inhibitors include tofacitinib, an oral medication used to treat ulcerative colitis. It can cause difficulty breathing or swallowing, rash, hives, swollen face (including the mouth) or swollen hands and feet, headaches, runny nose, nausea, and joint pain.[115]

ACKNOWLEDGMENTS

This book began in complete isolation. I did not tell anyone about it, and I began the arduous chore with virtually no guidance about how to proceed. After finally producing a manuscript that I thought was ready, I began looking for a publisher—only then realizing how difficult it was if you're new to this game. I want to thank the incredible team at Scribe Media for believing in my book and taking me on. Specifically, I would like to thank my publishing managers, Emmy and Meg, and my editor, Mark. Thank y'all for bearing with me!

To Mark Holleman, a great man and mentor who allowed me to use an empty office where I worked on this book at nights and on weekends. I am fortunate to have two wonderful siblings, Elizabeth and Henry, who always keep things fun. To my parents, Robert and Carrie, who got more than they bargained for with me. I cannot express how grateful I am for all y'all have done for me.

To my future wife and children: I don't know you yet, but I wrote this book, and launched my health business, for you. Finally, I am extremely blessed to have a merciful God who continues to give me second chances at life.

NOTES

1   Hendrik Van den Berg, *Economic Growth and Development*, 2nd ed. (World Scientific, 2012), 82.

2   Hendrik Van den Berg, *Economic Growth and Development*, 2nd ed. (World Scientific, 2012), 84.

3   Russell Roberts, *Life in Colonial America* (Mitchell Lane, 2007), 32.

4   John Komlos, "On the Biological Standard of Living of Eighteenth-Century Americans: Taller, Richer, Healthier," Munich Discussion Paper No. 2003-9 (Department of Economics, University of Munich, July 2003), 1-45, https://doi.org/10.5282/ubm/epub.53.

5   Kathleen B. Watson et al., "Trends in Multiple Chronic Conditions Among US Adults, by Life Stage, Behavioral Risk Factor Surveillance System, 2013-2023," *Preventing Chronic Disease* 22 (April 17, 2025): 1-4, 240539, http://dx.doi.org/10.5888/pcd22.240539.

6   "IBD Facts and Stats," US Centers for Disease Control and Prevention, June 21, 2024, https://www.cdc.gov/inflammatory-bowel-disease/php/facts-stats/index.html.

7   Tufts University Diet and Nutrition Letter, "Food for Thought," Tufts University.

8   Anne B. Martin et al., "National Health Expenditures in 2023: Faster Growth as Insurance Coverage and Utilization Increased," *Health Affairs* 44, no. 1 (2025): 12-13, https://doi.org/10.1377/hlthaff.2024.01375.

9   Anne B. Martin et al., "National Health Expenditures in 2023: Faster Growth as Insurance Coverage and Utilization Increased," *Health Affairs* 44, no. 1 (2025): 12-13, https://doi.org/10.1377/hlthaff.2024.01375.

10 Christine Buttorff et al., *Multiple Chronic Conditions in the United States* (Rand, 2017), 1, 6, https://www.rand.org/content/dam/rand/pubs/tools/TL200/TL221/RAND_TL221.pdf?%3E.

11 "Trend to Watch: The Percentage of Americans Taking Four or More Prescription Medications Daily Continues to Rise," CivicScience, February 18, 2025, https://civicscience.com/trend-to-watch-the-percentage-of-americans-taking-four-or-more-prescription-medications-daily-continues-to-rise/.

12 Karma Yeshi et al., "Current Treatments, Emerging Therapeutics, and Natural Remedies for Inflammatory Bowel Disease," *Molecules* 29, no. 16 (2024): 1, 3954, https://doi.org/10.3390/molecules29163954.

13 Farhad Mehrtash, "Sustained Crohn's Disease Remission with an Exclusive Elemental and Exclusion Diet: A Case Report," *Gastrointestinal Disorders* 3, no. 3 (2021): 130, https://doi.org/10.3390/gidisord3030014.

14   Farhad Mehrtash, "Sustained Crohn's Disease Remission with an Exclusive Elemental and Exclusion Diet: A Case Report," *Gastrointestinal Disorders* 3, no. 3 (2021): 129, https://doi.org/10.3390/gidisord3030014.

15   Karma Yeshi et al., "Current Treatments, Emerging Therapeutics, and Natural Remedies for Inflammatory Bowel Disease," *Molecules* 29, no. 16 (2024): 2, 3954, https://doi.org/10.3390/molecules29163954.

16   Rakesh K. Sindhu et al., "Crohn's Disease: Symptoms, Diagnosis, Management by Medical and Alternative Treatment," *Pharmaceutical Sciences Asia* 48, no. 3 (2021): 206, https://doi.org/10.29090/psa.2021.03.20.065.

17   Giacomo Caio et al., "Nutritional Treatment in Crohn's Disease," *Nutrients* 13, no. 5 (2021): 2, 1628, https://doi.org/10.3390/nu13051628.

18   Dermot P. B. McGovern et al., "Genetics of Inflammatory Bowel Diseases," *Gastroenterology* 149, no. 5 (2015): 1169, https://doi.org/10.1053/j.gastro.2015.08.001.

19   Daniele Piovani et al., "Environmental Risk Factors for Inflammatory Bowel Diseases: An Umbrella Review of Meta-Analyses," *Gastroenterology* 157, no. 3 (2019): 649, https://doi.org/10.1053/j.gastro.2019.04.016.

20   Daniele Piovani et al., "Environmental Risk Factors for Inflammatory Bowel Diseases: An Umbrella Review of Meta-Analyses," *Gastroenterology* 157, no. 3 (2019): 649–651, https://doi.org/10.1053/j.gastro.2019.04.016.

21   Daniele Piovani et al., "Environmental Risk Factors for Inflammatory Bowel Diseases: An Umbrella Review of Meta-Analyses," *Gastroenterology* 157, no. 3 (2019): 649, https://doi.org/10.1053/j.gastro.2019.04.016.

22   Daniele Piovani et al., "Environmental Risk Factors for Inflammatory Bowel Diseases: An Umbrella Review of Meta-Analyses," *Gastroenterology* 157, no. 3 (2019): 653, https://doi.org/10.1053/j.gastro.2019.04.016.

23   Rui Wang et al., "Global, Regional and National Burden of Inflammatory Bowel Disease in 204 Countries and Territories from 1990 to 2019: A Systematic Analysis Based on the Global Burden of Disease Study 2019," *BMJ Open* 13, no. 3 (2023): 2–8, e065186, https://doi.org/10.1136/bmjopen-2022-065186.

24   Gustavo Zarini et al., "Clinical and Anthropometric Improvements with a Tailored Dietary Approach in Pediatric Crohn's Disease," *Alternative Therapies in Health and Medicine* 27, no. S1 (2021): 190, https://pubmed.ncbi.nlm.nih.gov/33711815/.

25   Farhad Mehrtash, "Sustained Crohn's Disease Remission with an Exclusive Elemental and Exclusion Diet: A Case Report," *Gastrointestinal Disorders* 3, no. 3 (2021): 129, https://doi.org/10.3390/gidisord3030014.

26   Farhad Mehrtash, "Sustained Crohn's Disease Remission with an Exclusive Elemental and Exclusion Diet: A Case Report," *Gastrointestinal Disorders* 3, no. 3 (2021): 133, https://doi.org/10.3390/gidisord3030014.

27   Heather Mac Donald, "The Corruption of Medicine: Guardians of the Profession Discard Merit in Order to Alter the Demographics of Their Field," *City Journal*, Summer 2022, https://www.city-journal.org/article/the-corruption-of-medicine-2.

28   Haley Zynda, "The History of American Agriculture," *Ohio BEEF Cattle Letter* (blog), July 6, 2022, https://u.osu.edu/beef/2022/07/06/the-history-of-american-agriculture/.

29   Clare F. Donnellan et al., "Nutritional Management of Crohn's Disease," *Therapeutic Advances in Gastroenterology* 6, no. 3 (2013): 231, https://doi.org/10.1177/1756283X13477715.

30   Muna Shakhshir and Sa'ed H. Zyoud, "Global Research Trends on Diet and Nutrition in Crohn's Disease," *World Journal of Gastroenterology* 29, no. 20 (2023): 3204, https://doi.org/10.3748/wjg.v29.i20.3203.

31   Muna Shakhshir and Sa'ed H. Zyoud, "Global Research Trends on Diet and Nutrition in Crohn's Disease," *World Journal of Gastroenterology* 29, no. 20 (2023): 3205, https://doi.org/10.3748/wjg.v29.i20.3203.

32   Margaret Fosmoe, "George Gipp's Galloping Ghost," *Notre Dame Magazine*, December 14, 2020, https://magazine.nd.edu/stories/george-gipps-galloping-ghost/.

33   "Calvin Coolidge," White House Historical Association, accessed December 8, 2025, https://www.whitehousehistory.org/bios/calvin-coolidge.

34   Yuwei Zhang, "Colonoscopy: Unexpected Results from a Major Study, Is It Worth Doing?," *Epoch Times*, January 26, 2023, https://www.theepochtimes.com/health/colonoscopy-unexpected-results-from-a-major-study-is-it-worth-doing-5007390?welcomeuser=1.

35   Jordan S. Rubin, *Patient Heal Thyself: A Remarkable Health Program Combining Ancient Wisdom with Groundbreaking Clinical Research* (Freedom Press, 2003), 116.

36   John C. Warren, *Physical Education and the Preservation of Health* (William D. Ticknor and Company, 1846), 90.

37   Jack W. Berryman, "Exercise Is Medicine: A Historical Perspective," *Current Sports Medicine Reports* 9, no. 4 (2010): 197, https://doi.org/10.1249/JSR.0b013e3181e7d86d.

38   Jack W. Berryman, "Exercise Is Medicine: A Historical Perspective," *Current Sports Medicine Reports* 9, no. 4 (2010): 197, https://doi.org/10.1249/JSR.0b013e3181e7d86d.

39   Cintia Mayumi et al., "Abdominal Surgery in Crohn's Disease: Risk Factors for Complications," *Inflammatory Intestinal Diseases* 6, no. 1 (2021): 18, https://doi.org/10.1159/000510999.

40   Cintia Mayumi et al., "Abdominal Surgery in Crohn's Disease: Risk Factors for Complications," *Inflammatory Intestinal Diseases* 6, no. 1 (2021): 19, https://doi.org/10.1159/000510999.

41   Cintia Mayumi et al., "Abdominal Surgery in Crohn's Disease: Risk Factors for Complications," *Inflammatory Intestinal Diseases* 6, no. 1 (2021): 21, https://doi.org/10.1159/000510999.

42   Giacomo Caio et al., "Nutritional Treatment in Crohn's Disease," *Nutrients* 13, no. 5 (2021): 3, 1628, https://doi.org/10.3390/nu13051628.

43   Giacomo Caio et al., "Nutritional Treatment in Crohn's Disease," *Nutrients* 13, no. 5 (2021): 3, 1628, https://doi.org/10.3390/nu13051628.

44   Raymond Formanek Jr., "Updates: Remicade Approved for Children with Crohn's Disease," *FDA Consumer* 40, no. 4 (July –August 2006): 6.

45   Peter Doshi, "Revolving Doors: Board Memberships, Hedge Funds, and the FDA Chiefs Responsible for Regulating Industry," *BMJ* 385 (2024): 1, q975, https://doi.org/10.1136/bmj.q975.

46   Uma Mahadevan et al., "Infliximab and Semen Quality in Men with Inflammatory Bowel Disease," *Inflammatory Bowel Diseases* 11, no. 4 (2005): 395–399, https://doi.org/10.1097/01.MIB.0000164023.10848.c4.

47   Lauren Folgosa Cooley et al., "Anti-TNF Agents and Potential Effects on Male Fertility: Are Men Being Counseled?," *BMC Urology* 20, no. 1 (2020): 2–4, 111, https://doi.org/10.1186/s12894-020-00658-7.

48   Johnson & Johnson, "Proven Results," Remicade, accessed December 9, 2025, https://www.remicade.com/ulcerative-colitis/learn-about-remicade.html.

49   Jack W. Berryman, "Exercise Is Medicine: A Historical Perspective," *Current Sports Medicine Reports* 9, no. 4 (2010): 195, https://doi.org/10.1249/JSR.ob013e3181e7d86d.

50   Jack W. Berryman, "Exercise Is Medicine: A Historical Perspective," *Current Sports Medicine Reports* 9, no. 4 (2010): 195, https://doi.org/10.1249/JSR.ob013e3181e7d86d.

51   Jack W. Berryman, "Exercise Is Medicine: A Historical Perspective," *Current Sports Medicine Reports* 9, no. 4 (2010): 196, https://doi.org/10.1249/JSR.ob013e3181e7d86d.

52   William Buchan, *Domestic Medicine; Or, The Family Physician* (Balfour, Auld, and Smellie, 1769), 29.

53   Jack W. Berryman, "Exercise Is Medicine: A Historical Perspective," *Current Sports Medicine Reports* 9, no. 4 (2010): 198, https://doi.org/10.1249/JSR.ob013e3181e7d86d.

54   Naomi Lee et al., "Bone Loss in Crohn's Disease: Exercise as a Potential Countermeasure," *Inflammatory Bowel Diseases* 11, no. 12 (2005): 1109, https://doi.org/10.1097/01.MIB.0000192325.28168.08.

55   Naomi Lee et al., "Bone Loss in Crohn's Disease: Exercise as a Potential Countermeasure," *Inflammatory Bowel Diseases* 11, no. 12 (2005): 1108, https://doi.org/10.1097/01.MIB.0000192325.28168.08.

56   Naomi Lee et al., "Bone Loss in Crohn's Disease: Exercise as a Potential Countermeasure," *Inflammatory Bowel Diseases* 11, no. 12 (2005): 1115, https://doi.org/10.1097/01.MIB.0000192325.28168.08.

57   Anthony Samsel and Stephanie Seneff, "Glyphosate, Pathways to Modern Diseases II: Celiac Sprue and Gluten Intolerance," *Interdisciplinary Toxicology* 6, no. 4 (2013): 159–184, https://doi.org/10.2478/intox-2013-0026.

58   Anthony Samsel and Stephanie Seneff, "Glyphosate, Pathways to Modern Diseases II: Celiac Sprue and Gluten Intolerance," Interdisciplinary Toxicology 6, no. 4 (2013): 159–84.

59   Giacomo Caio et al., "Nutritional Treatment in Crohn's Disease," *Nutrients* 13, no. 5 (2021): 2–3, 1628, https://doi.org/10.3390/nu13051628.

60   Giacomo Caio et al., "Nutritional Treatment in Crohn's Disease," *Nutrients* 13, no. 5 (2021): 13, 1628, https://doi.org/10.3390/nu13051628.

61   Giacomo Caio et al., "Nutritional Treatment in Crohn's Disease," *Nutrients* 13, no. 5 (2021): 3, 1628, https://doi.org/10.3390/nu13051628.

62   Giacomo Caio et al., "Nutritional Treatment in Crohn's Disease," *Nutrients* 13, no. 5 (2021): 6, 1628, https://doi.org/10.3390/nu13051628.

63   Giacomo Caio et al., "Nutritional Treatment in Crohn's Disease," *Nutrients* 13, no. 5 (2021): 6, 1628, https://doi.org/10.3390/nu13051628.

64   Giacomo Caio et al., "Nutritional Treatment in Crohn's Disease," *Nutrients* 13, no. 5 (2021): 7, 1628, https://doi.org/10.3390/nu13051628.

65   Farhad Mehrtash, "Sustained Crohn's Disease Remission with an Exclusive Elemental and Exclusion Diet: A Case Report," *Gastrointestinal Disorders* 3, no. 3 (2021): 130, https://doi.org/10.3390/gidisord3030014.

66   Farhad Mehrtash, "Sustained Crohn's Disease Remission with an Exclusive Elemental and Exclusion Diet: A Case Report," *Gastrointestinal Disorders* 3, no. 3 (2021): 130, https://doi.org/10.3390/gidisord3030014.

67   Barbara De Conno et al., "Nutraceuticals and Diet Supplements in Crohn's Disease: A General Overview of the Most Promising Approaches in the Clinic," *Foods* 11, no. 7 (2022): 2, 1044, https://doi.org/10.3390/foods11071044.

68 Barbara De Conno et al., "Nutraceuticals and Diet Supplements in Crohn's Disease: A General Overview of the Most Promising Approaches in the Clinic," *Foods* 11, no. 7 (2022): 2, 1044, https://doi.org/10.3390/foods11071044.

69 Barbara De Conno et al., "Nutraceuticals and Diet Supplements in Crohn's Disease: A General Overview of the Most Promising Approaches in the Clinic," *Foods* 11, no. 7 (2022): 2, 1044, https://doi.org/10.3390/foods11071044.

70 Barbara De Conno et al., "Nutraceuticals and Diet Supplements in Crohn's Disease: A General Overview of the Most Promising Approaches in the Clinic," *Foods* 11, no. 7 (2022): 8, 1044, https://doi.org/10.3390/foods11071044.

71 Barbara De Conno et al., "Nutraceuticals and Diet Supplements in Crohn's Disease: A General Overview of the Most Promising Approaches in the Clinic," *Foods* 11, no. 7 (2022): 9, 1044, https://doi.org/10.3390/foods11071044.

72 Barbara De Conno et al., "Nutraceuticals and Diet Supplements in Crohn's Disease: A General Overview of the Most Promising Approaches in the Clinic," *Foods* 11, no. 7 (2022): 10, 1044, https://doi.org/10.3390/foods11071044.

73 Charlotte M. Verburgt et al., "Nutritional Therapy Strategies in Pediatric Crohn's Disease," *Nutrients* 13, no. 1 (2021): 4, 212, https://doi.org/10.3390/nu13010212.

74 Giacomo Caio et al., "Nutritional Treatment in Crohn's Disease," Nutrients 13, no. 5 (2021): 1628, https://doi.org/10.3390/nu13051628.

75 Giacomo Caio et al., "Nutritional Treatment in Crohn's Disease," Nutrients 13, no. 5 (2021): 1628, https://doi.org/10.3390/nu13051628.

76 Jason Nasser et al., "Elemental Diet as a Therapeutic Modality: A Comprehensive Review," *Digestive Diseases and Sciences* 69, no. 9 (2024): 3344, https://doi.org/10.1007/s10620-024-08543-1.

77 Jason Nasser et al., "Elemental Diet as a Therapeutic Modality: A Comprehensive Review," *Digestive Diseases and Sciences* 69, no. 9 (2024): 3344–3345, https://doi.org/10.1007/s10620-024-08543-1.

78 Jason Nasser et al., "Elemental Diet as a Therapeutic Modality: A Comprehensive Review," *Digestive Diseases and Sciences* 69, no. 9 (2024): 3344, https://doi.org/10.1007/s10620-024-08543-1.

79 Jason Nasser et al., "Elemental Diet as a Therapeutic Modality: A Comprehensive Review," *Digestive Diseases and Sciences* 69, no. 9 (2024): 3349, https://doi.org/10.1007/s10620-024-08543-1.

80 Jason Nasser et al., "Elemental Diet as a Therapeutic Modality: A Comprehensive Review," *Digestive Diseases and Sciences* 69, no. 9 (2024): 3349, https://doi.org/10.1007/s10620-024-08543-1.

81 Blanca Ferreiro et al., "Clinical and Nutritional Impact of a Semi-Elemental Hydrolyzed Whey Protein Diet in Patients with Active Crohn's Disease: A Prospective Observational Study," *Nutrients* 13, no. 10 (2021): 7, 3623, https://doi.org/10.3390/nu13103623.

82 Blanca Ferreiro et al., "Clinical and Nutritional Impact of a Semi-Elemental Hydrolyzed Whey Protein Diet in Patients with Active Crohn's Disease: A Prospective Observational Study," *Nutrients* 13, no. 10 (2021): 9, 3623, https://doi.org/10.3390/nu13103623.

83 Farhad Mehrtash, "Sustained Crohn's Disease Remission with an Exclusive Elemental and Exclusion Diet: A Case Report," *Gastrointestinal Disorders* 3, no. 3 (2021): 131, https://doi.org/10.3390/gidisord3030014.

84 Farhad Mehrtash, "Sustained Crohn's Disease Remission with an Exclusive Elemental and Exclusion Diet: A Case Report," *Gastrointestinal Disorders* 3, no. 3 (2021): 134, https://doi.org/10.3390/gidisord3030014.

85   Gustavo Zarini et al., "Clinical and Anthropometric Improvements with a Tailored Dietary Approach in Pediatric Crohn's Disease," *Alternative Therapies in Health and Medicine* 27, no. S1 (2021): 190–194, https://pubmed.ncbi.nlm.nih.gov/33711815/.

86   Gustavo Zarini et al., "Clinical and Anthropometric Improvements with a Tailored Dietary Approach in Pediatric Crohn's Disease," *Alternative Therapies in Health and Medicine* 27, no. S1 (2021): 191, https://pubmed.ncbi.nlm.nih.gov/33711815/.

87   "Omeprazole (Oral Route)," Mayo Clinic, last modified November 30, 2025, https://www.mayoclinic.org/drugs-supplements/omeprazole-oral-route/description/drg-20066836.

88   Gustavo Zarini et al., "Clinical and Anthropometric Improvements with a Tailored Dietary Approach in Pediatric Crohn's Disease," *Alternative Therapies in Health and Medicine* 27, no. S1 (2021): 190, https://pubmed.ncbi.nlm.nih.gov/33711815/.

89   Gustavo Zarini et al., "Clinical and Anthropometric Improvements with a Tailored Dietary Approach in Pediatric Crohn's Disease," *Alternative Therapies in Health and Medicine* 27, no. S1 (2021): 191, https://pubmed.ncbi.nlm.nih.gov/33711815/.

90   Gustavo Zarini et al., "Clinical and Anthropometric Improvements with a Tailored Dietary Approach in Pediatric Crohn's Disease," *Alternative Therapies in Health and Medicine* 27, no. S1 (2021): 191, https://pubmed.ncbi.nlm.nih.gov/33711815/.

91   Gustavo Zarini et al., "Clinical and Anthropometric Improvements with a Tailored Dietary Approach in Pediatric Crohn's Disease," *Alternative Therapies in Health and Medicine* 27, no. S1 (2021): 191, https://pubmed.ncbi.nlm.nih.gov/33711815/.

92   Gustavo Zarini et al., "Clinical and Anthropometric Improvements with a Tailored Dietary Approach in Pediatric Crohn's Disease," *Alternative Therapies in Health and Medicine* 27, no. S1 (2021): 191, https://pubmed.ncbi.nlm.nih.gov/33711815/.

93   Gustavo Zarini et al., "Clinical and Anthropometric Improvements with a Tailored Dietary Approach in Pediatric Crohn's Disease," *Alternative Therapies in Health and Medicine* 27, no. S1 (2021): 191, https://pubmed.ncbi.nlm.nih.gov/33711815/.

94   Gustavo Zarini et al., "Clinical and Anthropometric Improvements with a Tailored Dietary Approach in Pediatric Crohn's Disease," *Alternative Therapies in Health and Medicine* 27, no. S1 (2021): 191–192, https://pubmed.ncbi.nlm.nih.gov/33711815/.

95   Gustavo Zarini et al., "Clinical and Anthropometric Improvements with a Tailored Dietary Approach in Pediatric Crohn's Disease," *Alternative Therapies in Health and Medicine* 27, no. S1 (2021): 192, https://pubmed.ncbi.nlm.nih.gov/33711815/.

96   Jini Patel Thompson, *Listen to Your Gut: The Complete Natural Healing Program for IBS and IBD*, rev. and expanded ed. (Caramal Publishing, 2012), 267.

97   Jini Patel Thompson, *Listen to Your Gut: The Complete Natural Healing Program for IBS and IBD*, rev. and expanded ed. (Caramal Publishing, 2012), 270–272.

98   Jini Patel Thompson, *Listen to Your Gut: The Complete Natural Healing Program for IBS and IBD*, rev. and expanded ed. (Caramal Publishing, 2012), 273–275.

99   Paul C. Bernhardt et al., "Testosterone Changes During Vicarious Experiences of Winning and Losing Among Fans at Sporting Events," *Physiology and Behavior* 65, no. 1 (1998): 59–62, https://doi.org/10.1016/S0031-9384(98)00147-4.

100 Jini Patel Thompson, Listen to Your Gut: The Complete Natural Healing Program for IBS & IBD, rev. ed. (Vancouver, BC: Caramal Publishing, 2006), 318.

101 AbbVie, "U.S. FDA Approves RINVOQ (upadacitinib) as a Once-Daily Pill for Moderately to Severely Active Crohn's Disease in Adults," news release, May 18, 2023, https://news.abbvie.com/2023-05-18-U-S-FDA-Approves-RINVOQ-R-upadacitinib-as-a-Once-Daily-Pill-for-Moderately-to-Severely-Active-Crohns-Disease-in-Adults.

102 AbbVie, "About RINVOQ," Rinvoq, accessed December 9, 2025, https://www.rinvoq.com/.

103 Abbvie, *Skyrizi Label* (US Food and Drug Administration, 2024), 1.

104 Abbvie, *Skyrizi Label* (US Food and Drug Administration, 2019), 7.

105 Karma Yeshi et al., "Current Treatments, Emerging Therapeutics, and Natural Remedies for Inflammatory Bowel Disease," *Molecules* 29, no. 16 (2024): 1, 3954, https://doi.org/10.3390/molecules29163954.

106 Karma Yeshi et al., "Current Treatments, Emerging Therapeutics, and Natural Remedies for Inflammatory Bowel Disease," *Molecules* 29, no. 16 (2024): 2, 3954, https://doi.org/10.3390/molecules29163954.

107 Karma Yeshi et al., "Current Treatments, Emerging Therapeutics, and Natural Remedies for Inflammatory Bowel Disease," *Molecules* 29, no. 16 (2024): 2, 3954, https://doi.org/10.3390/molecules29163954.

108 Karma Yeshi et al., "Current Treatments, Emerging Therapeutics, and Natural Remedies for Inflammatory Bowel Disease," *Molecules* 29, no. 16 (2024): 3, 3954, https://doi.org/10.3390/molecules29163954.

109 Karma Yeshi et al., "Current Treatments, Emerging Therapeutics, and Natural Remedies for Inflammatory Bowel Disease," *Molecules* 29, no. 16 (2024): 4, 3954, https://doi.org/10.3390/molecules29163954.

110 Karma Yeshi et al., "Current Treatments, Emerging Therapeutics, and Natural Remedies for Inflammatory Bowel Disease," *Molecules* 29, no. 16 (2024): 4, 3954, https://doi.org/10.3390/molecules29163954.

111 Karma Yeshi et al., "Current Treatments, Emerging Therapeutics, and Natural Remedies for Inflammatory Bowel Disease," *Molecules* 29, no. 16 (2024): 4, 3954, https://doi.org/10.3390/molecules29163954.

112 Karma Yeshi et al., "Current Treatments, Emerging Therapeutics, and Natural Remedies for Inflammatory Bowel Disease," *Molecules* 29, no. 16 (2024): 7, 3954, https://doi.org/10.3390/molecules29163954.

113 Karma Yeshi et al., "Current Treatments, Emerging Therapeutics, and Natural Remedies for Inflammatory Bowel Disease," *Molecules* 29, no. 16 (2024): 4, 3954, https://doi.org/10.3390/molecules29163954.

114 Karma Yeshi et al., "Current Treatments, Emerging Therapeutics, and Natural Remedies for Inflammatory Bowel Disease," *Molecules* 29, no. 16 (2024): 7, 3954, https://doi.org/10.3390/molecules29163954.

115 Karma Yeshi et al., "Current Treatments, Emerging Therapeutics, and Natural Remedies for Inflammatory Bowel Disease," *Molecules* 29, no. 16 (2024): 5, 3954, https://doi.org/10.3390/molecules29163954.

www.ingramcontent.com/pod-product-compliance
Lightning Source LLC
Chambersburg PA
CBHW032032050726

47590CB00006B/2385